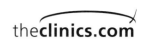

CHILD AND ADOLESCENT PSYCHIATRIC CLINICS OF NORTH AMERICA

Evidence-Based Practice, Part II:
Effecting Change

GUEST EDITORS
Barbara J. Burns, PhD, and
Kimberly Eaton Hoagwood, PhD

CONSULTING EDITOR
Melvin Lewis, MBBS, FRCPsych, DCH

April 2005 • Volume 14 • Number 2

SAUNDERS

An Imprint of Elsevier, Inc.
PHILADELPHIA   LONDON   TORONTO   MONTREAL   SYDNEY   TOKYO

W.B. SAUNDERS COMPANY
A Division of Elsevier Inc.

The Curtis Center • Independence Square West • Philadelphia, Pennsylvania 19106

http://www.theclinics.com

CHILD AND ADOLESCENT PSYCHIATRIC CLINICS
OF NORTH AMERICA Volume 14, Number 2
April 2005 ISSN 1056-4993
Editor: Sarah E. Barth ISBN 1-4160-2672-X

Reprints: For copies of 100 or more, of articles in this publication, please contact the Commercial Reprints Department, Elsevier Inc., 360 Park Avenue South, New York, New York 10010-1710. Tel. (212) 633-3813 Fax: (212) 462-1935 email: reprints@elsevier.com

The ideas and opinions expressed in *Child and Adolescent Psychiatric Clinics of North America* do not necessarily reflect those of the Publisher. The Publisher does not assume any responsibility for any injury and/or damage to persons or property arising out of or related to any use of the material contained in this periodical. The reader is advised to check the appropriate medical literature and the product information currently provided by the manufacturer of each drug to be administered to verify the dosage, the method and duration of administration, or contraindications. It is the responsibility of the treating physician or other health care professional, relying on independent experience and knowledge of the patient, to determine drug dosages and the best treatment for the patient. Mention of any product in this issue should not be construed as endorsement by the contributors, editors, or the Publisher of the product or manufacturers' claims.

Child and Adolescent Psychiatric Clinics of North America (ISSN 1056-4993) is published quarterly by W.B. Saunders Company. Corporate and editorial offices: The Curtis Center, Independence Square West, Philadelphia, PA 19106-3399. Accounting and circulation offices: 6277 Sea Harbor Drive, Orlando, FL 32887-4800. Periodicals postage paid at Orlando, FL 32862, and additional mailing offices. Subscription prices are $175.00 per year (US individuals), $265.00 per year (US institutions), $200.00 per year (Canadian individuals), $314.00 per year (Canadian institutions), $220.00 per year (foreign individuals), and $314.00 per year (foreign institutions). Foreign air speed delivery is included in all *Clinics* subscription prices. All prices are subject to change without notice. POSTMASTER: Send address changes to *Child and Adolescent Psychiatric Clinics of North America*, W.B. Saunders Company, Periodicals Fulfillment, Orlando, FL 32887-4800. **Customer Service: 1-800-654-2452 (US).** From outside the US, call 1-407-345-4000. E-mail: hhspcs@harcourt.com.

Child and Adolescent Psychiatric Clinics of North America is covered in *Index Medicus, ISI, SSCI, Research Alert, Social Search, Current Contents,* and *EMBASE/Excerpta Medica.*

Printed in the United States of America.

CONSULTING EDITOR

MELVIN LEWIS, MBBS, FRCPsych, DCH, Professor Emeritus, Senior Research Scientist, Yale Child Study Center, Yale University School of Medicine, New Haven, Connecticut

GUEST EDITORS

BARBARA J. BURNS, PhD, Professor of Medical Psychology, Services Effectiveness Research Program, Department of Psychiatry and Behavioral Sciences, Duke University School of Medicine, Durham, North Carolina

KIMBERLY EATON HOAGWOOD, PhD, Professor of Clinical Psychology and Psychiatry, Department of Child Psychiatry, Columbia University; Director of Child and Adolescent Services Research, Office of Mental Health, State of New York, New York, New York

CONTRIBUTORS

GREGORY A. AARONS, PhD, Research Scientist, Child and Adolescent Services Research Center, San Diego; Assistant Clinical Professor, Department of Psychiatry; Associate Project Scientist, Department of Psychology, University of California–San Diego, School of Medicine, La Jolla, California

LEONARD BICKMAN, PhD, Director, Center for Evaluation and Program Improvement, Peabody College; Associate Dean of Research, Peabody College; Professor of Psychology and Public Policy, Department of Psychology and Human Development, Vanderbilt University, Nashville, Tennessee

ALFIEE BRELAND-NOBLE, PhD, Duke Pediatric EBM Seminar Team, Department of Psychiatry and Behavioral Sciences, Duke Child and Family Study Center, Duke University Medical Center, Durham, North Carolina

DAVID A. CHAMBERS, PhD, Chief, Dissemination and Implementation Research Program, National Institute of Mental Health, Rockville, Maryland

BRUCE F. CHORPITA, PhD, Department of Psychology, University of Hawaii at Manoa, Honolulu, Hawaii

ALLAN CHRISMAN, MD, Duke Pediatric EBM Seminar Team, Department of Psychiatry and Behavioral Sciences, Duke Child and Family Study Center, Duke University Medical Center, Durham, North Carolina

KELLY CLOUSE, MD, Duke Pediatric EBM Seminar Team, Department of Psychiatry and Behavioral Sciences, Duke Child and Family Study Center, Duke University Medical Center, Durham, North Carolina

RICHARD D'ALLI, MD, Duke Pediatric EBM Seminar Team, Department of Psychiatry and Behavioral Sciences, Duke Child and Family Study Center, Duke University Medical Center, Durham, North Carolina

ERIC L. DALEIDEN, PhD, Child and Adolescent Mental Health Division, Hawaii Department of Health; Department of Psychiatry, John A. Burns School of Medicine, University of Hawaii at Manoa, Honolulu, Hawaii

MINA K. DULCAN, MD, Head, Child and Adolescent Psychiatry, Osterman Professor of Child Psychiatry, Children's Memorial Hospital; Professor of Psychiatry and Behavioral Sciences and Pediatrics, Northwestern University, Feinberg School of Medicine, Chicago, Illinois

HELEN EGGER, MD, Duke Pediatric EBM Seminar Team, Department of Psychiatry and Behavioral Sciences, Duke Child and Family Study Center, Duke University Medical Center, Durham, North Carolina

LAURIE M. FLYNN, Director, Carmel Hill Center for Early Diagnosis and Treatment, Division of Child and Adolescent Psychiatry, Columbia University, New York, New York

EILEEN FRANCO, MPH, Project Manager, National Evaluation of the Comprehensive Community Mental Health Services for Children and Their Families Program, ORC Macro, Atlanta, Georgia

PAT GAMMON, PhD, Duke Pediatric EBM Seminar Team, Department of Psychiatry and Behavioral Sciences, Duke Child and Family Study Center, Duke University Medical Center, Durham, North Carolina

MARTA GAZZOLA, MD, Duke Pediatric EBM Seminar Team, Department of Psychiatry and Behavioral Sciences, Duke Child and Family Study Center, Duke University Medical Center, Durham, North Carolina

PAUL GORMAN, EdD, Director, West Institute at the New Hampshire-Dartmouth Psychiatric Research Center, Dartmouth Medical School, Lebanon, New Hampshire

ENITH E. HICKMAN, MPH, Social Science Research Analyst, Centers for Medicare & Medicaid Services, Baltimore, Maryland

ANNE LIN, MD, Duke Pediatric EBM Seminar Team, Department of Psychiatry and Behavioral Sciences, Duke Child and Family Study Center, Duke University Medical Center, Durham, North Carolina

DAVID W. LYNDE, MSW, LICSW, Training Manager, West Institute at the New Hampshire-Dartmouth Psychiatric Research Center, Dartmouth Medical School, Lebanon, New Hampshire

JOHN S. MARCH, MD, MPH, Duke Pediatric EBM Seminar Team, Department of Psychiatry and Behavioral Sciences, Duke Child and Family Study Center, Duke University Medical Center, Durham, North Carolina

CHRISTIAN MAURO, PhD, Duke Pediatric EBM Seminar Team, Department of Psychiatry and Behavioral Sciences, Duke Child and Family Study Center, Duke University Medical Center, Durham, North Carolina

MARY McBRIDE, PhD, Assistant Director, Clackamas County Mental Health, Oregon City, Oregon

AASIM RANA, MD, Duke Pediatric EBM Seminar Team, Department of Psychiatry and Behavioral Sciences, Duke Child and Family Study Center, Duke University Medical Center, Durham, North Carolina

HIMABINDU RAVI, MD, Duke Pediatric EBM Seminar Team, Department of Psychiatry and Behavioral Sciences, Duke Child and Family Study Center, Duke University Medical Center, Durham, North Carolina

MANUEL RIEMER, MS, Graduate Student, Department of Psychology and Human Development, Vanderbilt University, Nashville, Tennessee

HEATHER RINGEISEN, PhD, Chief, Child and Adolescent Services Research Program, National Institute of Mental Health, Rockville, Maryland

JULIE ROSOF-WILLIAMS, RN, MSN, Graduate Student, Department of Psychology and Human Development; Assistant to the Department of Pediatrics, Vanderbilt University School of Medicine, Nashville, Tennessee

ROBIN E. SOLER, PhD, Technical Director, National Evaluation of the Comprehensive Community Mental Health Services for Children and Their Families Program, ORC Macro, Atlanta, Georgia

MADHANIKA SRIRAMA, MD, Duke Pediatric EBM Seminar Team, Department of Psychiatry and Behavioral Sciences, Duke Child and Family Study Center, Duke University Medical Center, Durham, North Carolina

HANSEN SU, MD, Duke Pediatric EBM Seminar Team, Department of Psychiatry and Behavioral Sciences, Duke Child and Family Study Center, Duke University Medical Center, Durham, North Carolina

GRACE THRALL, MD, Duke Pediatric EBM Seminar Team, Department of Psychiatry and Behavioral Sciences, Duke Child and Family Study Center, Duke University Medical Center, Durham, North Carolina

WILLIAM C. TORREY, MD, Medical Director, West Central Behavioral Health, Dartmouth-Hitchcock; Associate Professor of Psychiatry, West Institute at the New Hampshire-Dartmouth Psychiatric Research Center, Dartmouth Medical School, Lebanon, New Hampshire

POLLY VAN DE VELDE, MSW, Duke Pediatric EBM Seminar Team, Department of Psychiatry and Behavioral Sciences, Duke Child and Family Study Center, Duke University Medical Center, Durham, North Carolina

CONTENTS

> The focus on evidence-based practices has come to dominate discussions in medicine and mental health. Whereas professionals and providers focus on complex barriers to implementing and engaging administrative support, the realities for families are different. The mental health system in most communities is still fragmented and inaccessible, leaving parents overwhelmed and frustrated. To truly implement system reform, the practical needs and experiences of families must become a key strategic element.

> Most aspiring child mental health professionals would support the premise that clinical practice should have a scientific foundation. Why, then, is the implementation of evidence-based practice in child and adolescent psychiatry so difficult? Considering the multiple stakeholders in clinical work, impediments are not surprising. Practitioner delays in implementation of research findings are common to all specialties of medicine. This article outlines the barriers to implementation of evidence-based practice and suggests changes to motivate and enable clinicians to use evidence-based practices.

the strength of the evidence but also on the processes and tools that are necessary for clinicians to continually upgrade their knowledge and skills for those problems encountered in daily practice. This article, authored by members of the Duke Pediatric Psychiatry EBM Seminar Team, (1) describes EBM as applied to the training of child and adolescent psychiatrists in the Division of Child and Adolescent Psychiatry, Department of Psychiatry at Duke University Medical Center; (2) presents a simplified discussion of EBM as a technology for training and patient care; (3) discusses the basic principles and procedures for teaching EBM in the setting of a multidisciplinary training program; and (4) briefly mentions two training and research initiatives that are furthered by incorporating EBM.

The National Implementing Evidence-Based Practice Project is an ongoing effort to promote the implementation of effective practices for adults who have severe mental illnesses. The project members designed and developed integrated packages of materials and services to help practice sites implement evidence-based practices and is field-testing the approach in eight states. These implementations are being evaluated carefully to learn how to make the technology transfer process more efficient in the future. This article describes the project and provides some early reflections on the implementation experience.

This article is a survey of many of the initiatives developed by federal and state agencies and foundations focusing on evidence-based mental health practices for children and adolescents. The article intends to show the tremendous interest in the development, dissemination, and implementation of evidence-based practice in child and adolescent mental health that is held by a wide variety of agencies and organizations. Several "next steps" for the field are suggested that might be developed in a subsequent series of initiatives. These steps include a better understanding of dissemination and implementation processes, increased clarity around definitions and terms, increased efforts to build infrastructure and support policy change, and the potential for an aggregation of data already gathered on the implementation of evidence-based practices.

FORTHCOMING ISSUES

RECENT ISSUES

THE CLINICS ARE NOW AVAILABLE ONLINE!

Access your subscription at:
http://www.theclinics.com

ELSEVIER
SAUNDERS

Child Adolesc Psychiatric Clin N Am
14 (2005) xiii

CHILD AND
ADOLESCENT
PSYCHIATRIC CLINICS
OF NORTH AMERICA

Foreword

Evidence-Based Practice, Part II: Effecting Change

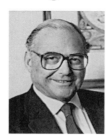

Melvin Lewis, MBBS, FRCPsych, DCH
Consulting Editor

The subject of evidence-based practice in child mental health care has now reached a level of sophistication that sets a high standard in child psychiatry practice.

The nature of the "evidence" for evidence-based practice is intelligently discussed at the outset of this two-part series of *Child and Adolescent Psychiatric Clinics of North America*. Part I (published in October 2004) and Part II together comprise a comprehensive review of evidence-based practice. Part I contains updates in the following areas: intensive home-based and community interventions, school-based interventions, engaging families, and psychotropic medications. Part II includes a series of articles on perspectives about evidence-based practices and strategies for moving them into clinical practice.

I am very grateful to the co-guest editors, Barbara J. Burns and Kimberly Eaton Hoagwood, and the outstanding group of authors they have recruited for this issue. This issue is an important statement of where we stand in evidence-based treatment and where we might go in the future. This is an important issue that should be read by all clinicians who treat children and adolescents.

Melvin Lewis, MBBS, FRCPsych, DCH
Yale University Child Study Center
230 South Frontgate Road
New Haven, CT 06520, USA
E-mail address: Melvin.lewis@yale.edu

doi:10.1016/j.chc.2005.01.001

CHILD AND
ADOLESCENT
PSYCHIATRIC CLINICS
OF NORTH AMERICA

ELSEVIER
SAUNDERS

Child Adolesc Psychiatric Clin N Am
14 (2005) xv–xvii

Preface

Evidence-Based Practice, Part II: Effecting Change

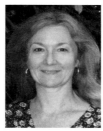

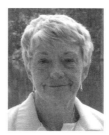

Kimberly Eaton Hoagwood, PhD   Barbara J. Burns, PhD
Guest Editors

This is the second installment of a two-part issue of the *Child and Adolescent Psychiatric Clinics of North America* focusing on evidence-based practices in child and adolescent mental health. The first issue provided a comprehensive update of the status of research findings for a range of treatment and service modalities, including psychotherapies, psychopharmacologies, home, school, and community interventions, and strategies for engaging families in mental health services. In addition, it drew attention to the constraints within the evidence base, especially with respect to understanding mechanisms of change. This second issue extends discussion about evidence-based practices for children by focusing on the challenges involved in implementing, disseminating, and sustaining these interventions in children's service delivery systems.

These issues together constitute the 5-year anniversary of the 1999 release of the Surgeon General's Report on Mental Health. That report represented an important turning point for children's mental health services by documenting the extensive evidence about the effectiveness of a range of mental health interventions for persons suffering from mental illness.

This second issue deepens the discussion by turning attention to the issues of context that out of necessity affect the implementation of evidence-based practices (EBPs). Context includes the attitudes, beliefs, and behaviors of multiple

doi:10.1016/j.chc.2004.11.001   *childpsych.theclinics.com* stakeholders who are touched by or involved in the adoption of new treatments or services. These stakeholders include families and their children, practitioners, clinicians, and administrators. Context also involves more macro-level organizational structures and their influence, including academic training centers, mental health agencies, and federal, state, and foundation agencies that set policies. Together these contextual factors influence the likelihood that EBPs—no matter how rigorously examined or effective—will be successfully incorporated into routine practice.

The articles in this issue address the range of context issues at both the stakeholder and organizational levels that affect implementation of EBPs. Because the majority of routine services delivered to children and adolescents with mental health problems have no evidence to support positive improvement for children, attention to ways of improving delivery through implementation of effective practices is arguably the most critical public health issue facing the mental health system.

In the first issue, we identified three social and scientific movements that lent support to the timeliness of this endeavor: research priority-setting by federal agencies targeted at strengthening the evidence base; federal and state policy initiatives focused on translating science to service; and increasing demand by advocates to improve access and quality of mental health care for children. The second issue delves deeply into the issues of what it takes to put these EBPs into place and how to effect sustained change.

The articles describing the views of stakeholders—especially families and practitioners—about evidence-based practices highlight the differences between the research-driven pursuit of increasingly nuanced questions versus the advocacy and practitioner-driven desire for answers and action. As the articles in this issue attest, these two pursuits are not mutually exclusive. The complexities involved in effecting change that touches the lives of families, advocates, and clinicians necessitates identification of a common ground.

Progress in bringing constructs from social, cognitive, and learning theories to bear on issues of clinician practice and provider attitudes offer important new directions for bridging basic and applied science. As the articles in this issue suggest, these advances are likely to lead to a better understanding of the processes of change that affect practitioners as well as organizations and systems.

Among the organizational structures that exert significant influence on clinician training are the academic training centers located throughout the country. New strategies for incorporating evidence-based medicine into ongoing physician training offer a model for promoting flexible, state-of-the-art training in EBPs. In addition, extensive efforts to disseminate specific EBPs in adult mental health through the National Implementing EBP Project offer important lessons for children's mental health about ways to incorporate multiple stakeholder perspectives, strengthen formal training, and incorporate outcome monitoring into all phases of the dissemination process. Finally, because a series of major federal, state, and foundation initiatives are shaping in profound ways the policy context for implementation of EBPs, a review of those major efforts is provided by federal science leaders on children's mental health and organizational research.

The issue ends with a description of two specific EBP implementation projects being undertaken in several states and systems. These projects are addressing the same issues—how to implement EBPs within systems—but from very different vantages. Both are pioneering efforts that are elucidating the challenges involved in these system-change efforts. The lessons learned from these projects offer importance guidance about the critical steps that must be taken to create effective and sustainable quality improvement efforts.

In conclusion, the articles in both issues represent a critical turning point in the evolution of children's mental health services. They document the significant scientific progress that has been achieved since the release of the Surgeon General's report. Even more importantly, they describe the challenges, strategies, and efforts of many committed individuals—from policymakers to advocates to researchers—to improve delivery of services to children and adolescents. The challenges are formidable; however, the goals are principled, and the potential impact of the changes is profound.

Having a scientifically validated knowledge base upon which to refocus treatment and service decisions is a necessary first step. However, as the articles in this issue demonstrate, the public health issues now facing families, practitioners, scientists, and policymakers are how best to incorporate new practices into systems and use the opportunity afforded by these changes to reform those systems. To do so requires a science on EBP implementation effectiveness that is grounded in practical wisdom. The articles in this issue reflect that melding.

Kimberly Eaton Hoagwood, PhD
Department of Child Psychiatry
Columbia University
1051 Riverside Drive #78
New York, NY 10031, USA
E-mail address: hoagwood@childpsych.columbia.edu

Barbara J. Burns, PhD
Department of Psychiatry and Behavioral Sciences
Duke University School of Medicine
Box 3454 DUMC
Durham, NC 27710, USA
E-mail address: bjb@geri.duke.edu

ELSEVIER
SAUNDERS

Child Adolesc Psychiatric Clin N Am
14 (2005) 217–224

CHILD AND
ADOLESCENT
PSYCHIATRIC CLINICS
OF NORTH AMERICA

Family Perspectives on Evidence-Based Practice

Laurie M. Flynn

*Carmel Hill Center for Early Diagnosis and Treatment, Division of Child and Adolescent Psychiatry,
Columbia University, 1775 Broadway, Suite 715, New York, NY 10019, USA*

"I'm not exactly sure what evidence-based practice (EBP) means, but I'm pretty sure we've never seen one!" That is what a parent who is a longtime friend said to me when I told her I was drafting this article and wanted to get input from families. Her comment, although a little sarcastic, reflects a reality: There is no agreed-upon definition for EBP. The term is widely used to describe all types of mental health programs and practices. So pervasive is the current focus on EBPs that some parents with whom I talked referred to this as "the latest buzz words," "a new trend for professionals," and "currently fashionable research." Comments like these point out the difference between what captures attention in the world of mental health care professionals and what seems important to parents. In this article, I draw on more than 20 years' experience of working with families and my own personal experiences with mental health services and providers to explore the concept of EBPs and the differing perspectives between professionals and the consumers and families they serve.

History of the evidence-based practice movement

Quality and accountability have become watchwords in health and mental health services. EBPs are a means to achieve both ends. To achieve the objective of accountable, high-quality services by implementing EBPs, however, much of what characterizes the current system must change [1]. The movement to demonstrate and document EBPs is one of the most powerful ideas in medicine. It was hailed as one of the most influential ideas of the year 2001 by the *New York Times Magazine*. The concept was developed in the wake of the managed care revolution of the 1990s and accompanying efforts to restrain the rise in health care costs. The idea was to create greater consistency in the treatment of major medical conditions and achieve better results by focusing on science-based interventions [2]. Reimbursement was linked in many health plans to the implementation of "practice guidelines." Providers were expected to justify their use

E-mail address: flynnl@childpsych.columbia.edu

of expensive or intensive interventions by referring to evidence of effectiveness as documented in peer-reviewed literature. Instead of relying on clinical experience or individual preference, practitioners were increasingly required to use treatment with a published record of successful outcomes.

Mental health care has a long history of being criticized for ineffective and inefficient practices. Treatment approaches have reflected strong belief systems rather than a strong research base. The range of providers and therapies used has not been subjected to rigorous review. It is not surprising that the research base on the efficacy of various interventions is weak in child mental health services. Only a few treatments have been reasonably well documented and studied, including the use of stimulants for attention deficit hyperactivity disorder, parent management strategies for behavior problems in young children, interpersonal therapies for depression, cognitive-behavioral therapies for children with anxiety, multisystemic therapy for aggressive and delinquent youth, and some emerging work on engagement techniques and certain school-based interventions [3].

In addition to the gaps in scientific research in children's mental health care is the lack of real standards for determining what constitutes an EBP. A professional consensus does not exist on when practices and interventions have reached readiness for community dissemination and can become the new standard of care [4]. Although the movement to provide treatment with an evidence base is widely praised, there is no clear agreement among professionals about what actually meets the definition of EBP. How much evidence is enough? How can we reconcile the results that emerge from controlled research settings with the "messy real world" conditions that characterize most service settings? EBPs must continue to evolve to meet these challenges. Research must address several critical issues, including strengthening the scientific underpinnings, practical matters of adaptation, and dissemination and problems of disparities in an uneven health care economy. To have maximum positive impact on mental health care for children and adolescents, however, the perspectives and priorities of families must be understood.

Evidence-based practices: the real world reality facing families

A recent review of the literature reveals that in child psychiatry and child mental health practice, there is an evidence base for only a small number of interventions [4]. We have much to learn to improve child mental health practice and treatment outcomes. Only in the past few years have researchers begun a systematic review of the many medications and therapies provided to children and adolescents. Although the National Institute of Mental Health has tripled its investment in research in child and adolescent mental disorders over the past 15 years, the field is still underdeveloped and underfunded. Diagnosis often is tentative, and most treatments are untested. It is common for a youngster to receive several different diagnoses over the first few years of mental health treatment.

The various disciplines that provide services for children and adolescents have widely varying training and often see the same symptoms as indicating different conditions, which causes parents understandable confusion and concern. The press has reported a fourfold increase in prescriptions of psychotropic drugs to children, but most of these medications never have been tested on children. Many of these drugs are prescribed "off label" and largely by non-psychiatrists. Parents frequently express discomfort with the gaps in knowledge and worry that their kids are being used as "guinea pigs" for research. "It's really hard to know what to believe," one mother told me recently. "The school and the doctor keep telling us to try medication but nobody seems to know if it will really work or what side effects might be. It's scary."

Younger and younger children are being diagnosed with mental health problems, even preschoolers in some cases. We still know almost nothing about the long-term effects of psychiatric medications on the developing brain. With several new drugs for attention deficit hyperactivity disorder and depression, how do parents determine what is best for their child? There is a dearth of evidence to guide their decision making; however, there are many opinions and controversy surrounding appropriate use of medications. A recent hearing held by the US Food and Drug Administration illustrated the heightened public concern about the widespread "off label" use of powerful psychotropic drugs. Prescription of these medications has increased exponentially during the past decade in an effort to treat a growing number of youngsters with a psychiatric diagnosis. Most doctors who prescribe such medications for children and adolescents are non-psychiatrists, however.

The situation with psychotherapy is no better. The intervention with the strongest evidence base is multisystemic therapy, and it has been tested mostly as an intervention with juvenile offenders [3]. There is promising work on cognitive behavior therapies with adolescents, but its applicability for younger children is not yet well known. Many clinicians believe that a combination of medication and psychotherapy is ideal, but few studies have been conducted to examine the combination, so little evidence exists to support this contention. In the real world of community providers, families are offered a range of unproven treatments with decidedly mixed results. Most often, families are referred for services to providers who describe their approach as "eclectic." Therapists are highly individual, and many are not certified in any particular technique. They do what they have been trained to do and rely on their instinct and ability to create a therapeutic alliance. Although a good rapport with a patient is a fundamental part of healing, it is not sufficient to relieve suffering.

Case vignette

A father I know recounted his family's frustrating experience over a 16-month period:

> When our son was 11 he began to have real problems, especially at school. We worked with the school counselor for several months. She believed the issue was adjustment to middle school, along with some academic problems. Then when things got worse, we went to a licensed social worker with an early adolescent

practice. She put our son in group therapy twice a week and told us working things out in the group and practicing problem solving was critical. But some of the kids in the group were a lot older than our son and several were court-committed juvenile delinquents. My boy actually told me he felt intimidated in the group and wanted to quit after only 2 months. Next we were referred to a clinical psychologist. He reviewed the case history and said we should begin family systems therapy. His theory was that we had screwed up family communication and inconsistent discipline. This meant all five of us were expected to spend Wednesday evenings in the doctor's office. It was a serious disruption in the family schedule and really added to my other child's anger. Plus my son also had weekly individual sessions. Each new professional seemed to have their own ideas and opinions and none of them spoke to the other people we had seen. I got really worried and angry about all the time and money we were spending yet things with my son were no better. The whole experience left me feeling very frustrated. How are you supposed to get good professional help when everyone has a different idea of what's wrong and how to fix it?

He did not realize it, but this father and his family were relatively lucky. At least they had the financial means to go to various mental health care providers. Around the country, thousands of families have problems with access to care. Coverage for mental health care in many insurance plans is limited, and managed care policies restrict choice and access to many providers. Because there are too few child psychiatrists, most youth with more severe symptoms are treated by a pediatrician or other primary care physician. Although they have good intentions, most of these family doctors have no training in psychiatric diagnosis and psychosocial or pharmacologic treatment. Not surprisingly, they may misdiagnose, undertreat, or overtreat, which further confuses a difficult situation and erodes parental trust in mental health care services.

Even in communities in which a full range of providers is available, there often are long waiting lists. The continuing lack of full parity in health insurance also means that mental health treatment is unaffordable for many families and children. Cost, not evidence, drives decisions about treatment for most parents. Differential insurance caps and co-pays make continuity of care difficult and expensive. Managed care restrictions mean that only a limited number of providers accept a case. Families report that it often takes many months of trying various services before they begin to understand what is wrong and what help they need. By then, thousands of dollars in coverage have been used up, with no real improvement in the youngster's functioning. In some cases, exhausted families are finally told they must give up legal custody of their child to access treatment through the public sector.

Families' perceptions of evidence-based practices

Parents are most focused on the practical issues in dealing with mental health services. The ideas behind EBPs seem remote from their daily experiences. The National Alliance for the Mentally Ill (NAMI), where I served for 16 years as executive director, has a growing number of members focused on child mental health policy and practice. Ken Duckworth, MD, NAMI's medical director, regularly convenes a telephone conference call with local and state leaders on issues of interest to families. On February 6, 2004, the group discussed EBPs in children's mental health. The lively 90-minute conversation elicited some key concerns and perspectives from parents with experience in the arena (D. Gruttadaro, MD, personal communication, 2004). A key observation was that although EBPs are a hot topic in policy and professional circles, the current health care system is not designed to serve children and adolescents with mental illnesses. Many parents are frankly doubtful that grafting EBPs onto a failed and fragmented system will succeed.

To some parents, the current controversy surrounding selective serotonin reuptake inhibitors and potential increased suicide risk, which recently led to another US Food and Drug Administration review of research evidence, makes clear that even government regulation is not a guarantee of quality. This has created considerable doubt in the one area that parents had previously trusted as an evidence-based treatment. As one parent I know said plaintively, "I'd like to use evidence-based psychiatry but I'm not sure how to find it." This remark mirrors the concerns for NAMI advocates who participated in the conference call from across the country. As informed consumers of mental health services, they are painfully aware that there is not much science yet on what works for kids. Even more disturbing is the shortage of licensed professionals to treat our children and adolescents. "Evidence-based practices aren't much help if there's nobody who will see my child," said one mother. In many communities, problems with access to care—any kind of care—have reached crisis proportions.

NAMI families reported that the cost of implementing EBPs is perceived as high, and local and state officials are facing budget shortfalls. Others observed that before EBP became a big focus, there was a lot of talk about "wraparound services" and systems of care for children. More than a decade after these ideas first entered the field, however, we do not see much improvement in the basic service structure. One participant asked, "How useful are all these good ideas if they never get implemented?" Meanwhile, the day-to-day burden of care and much of the case management still fall on parents.

When families talk about what they are looking for from evidence-based mental health services, the emphasis is on outcomes that go far beyond reduction of symptoms. Parents want to see their children improve in their school performance. They want treatment to help their kids relate better with friends and family. They also look to increased self-confidence and independence over the long-term as critical measures of treatment effectiveness. These are not the measures typically built into clinical research studies. It is clear that researchers should work more closely with parents and family advocacy organizations as they develop studies and define outcomes measures.

Another theme from the conference call was the importance of recognizing the impact of culture on treatment efficacy. Many parents of various ethnic and cultural backgrounds reported feeling unheard and even disrespected by mental health care professionals. Families play a crucial role in a fragmented system and are essential to recovery. A colleague recently commented, "Why haven't we found out more about how to work effectively with families? We're always reading about how families are part of their kids' problems, but not enough is known about the tremendous strength and endurance of families who deal every day with a disturbed child with almost no help."

Stigma is another burden borne by families, and its impact may be under-estimated. In a culture that still views children as a direct reflection of their families, parents whose children have behavioral disorders often feel ashamed and inadequate. Support for the families' role in treatment is frequently missing, or parents are relegated to serving as transportation to get their youngster to therapy. Some service providers focus attention exclusively on the child and ignore the needs and insights of parents. Others assume that most children with mental disorders come from "dysfunctional families" and that parents are the cause of a child's symptoms. These ideas and attitudes are readily perceived by parents, who often report feeling marginalized in their child's mental health care treatment.

Strong evidence exists from research with adults that caregiving is distressing and demanding. It can lead to impaired health and reduced quality of life for the caregiver. The additional burden of a professional community that is perceived as rejecting makes life even more difficult for parents. Many parents report feeling isolated and overwhelmed [5]. For parents who are trying to cope with an out-of-control child, upset or neglected siblings, ongoing financial and marital stress, and usually two full-time jobs, the reality is that negotiating with the child mental health and educational systems is a nightmare. Families repeatedly seek help in managing all these competing priorities and spend evenings and weekends searching for the latest evidence-based treatment solutions.

Schools often are another major battleground for parents. Several NAMI families noted that youth with untreated mental illness in middle and high schools are frequently viewed as delinquent and often end up in juvenile justice systems because of aggressive behaviors. Some parents reported that they and their ill child are told they must accept the special education programs offered—however inadequate—because the only alternative is referral to juvenile justice.

There is a real need to focus on school-based programs that are specific to kids with mental illnesses—not just kids with learning difficulties. Parents reported that traditional approaches frequently mix emotionally disturbed kids with kids who are coping with a wide range of other disabilities. "There is this one-size-fits-all mentality," noted one parent, "but not much is done beyond attempts at behavior modification through extensive use of 'time-outs.' What my daughter needs is more 'time-in' so she can learn how to interact and participate effectively in class."

The areas of highest interest to families as we pursue the work of defining and disseminating EBPs in child mental health include

- Improving family engagement
- Providing effective family education

- Supporting caregivers
- Medication decisions and managing side effects
- What works in psychotherapy
- Promoting independence and emancipation for severely disabled adolescents

Parents want to see improved school-based programs and worry that the presence of a mental disorder is the single greatest predictor of school dropout.

Beyond these specific concerns, there is overwhelming frustration with the slow pace of change in professional attitudes and practices. The effective partnership among researchers, leading professionals, and the family/consumer advocacy community that has defined standards of care in adult mental health must be built for children. The advocacy focus must be on expanding availability of effective outpatient treatment and creating a broader evidence base for service development. Until such a strategic partnership is in place, efforts at large-scale dissemination of EBPs will be difficult to achieve [6]. Accelerating the pace of community replication requires greater understanding of the realities of real world practice settings and policies.

Families must play a much greater role in identifying, developing, and promulgating EBPs. As individuals and through organized advocacy, families can facilitate research that speeds implementation of existing and new EBPs. Parents can be engaged in leading efforts to promote policies that support the adoption of EBPs through education and advocacy. They can influence provider behavior by acting as a "demand-side" for needed reform in practice. Families can help define an action research agenda that is motivating to policymakers, who often wonder about the results of programs they fund. These kinds of strategies generally have been relegated to a lower level of importance by professionals. Neglecting to ensure the "buy-in" of families and advocacy groups leads to poor results in the struggle for attention and resources, however. A more concrete and practical agenda for EBPs research and implementation could energize advocates and give families a real voice in this important scientific endeavor [7].

Acknowledgments

The author wishes to thank Ken Duckworth, MD, Darcy Gruttadaro, JD, and NAMI members who shared their experiences and reflections on evidence-based practices. Special thanks to Roisin O'Mara for her help with the manuscript.

References

[1] Goldman HH, Ganju V, Drake RE, Gorman P, Hogan M, Hyde PS, et al. Policy implications for implementing evidence-based practices. Psychiatr Serv 2001;52(12):1591–7.
[2] Haynes RB. What kind of evidence is it that evidence-based medicine advocates want health care providers and consumers to pay attention to? BMC Health Serv Res 2002;2(1):3.

[3] Hoagwood K, Burns BJ, Kiser L, Ringeisen H, Schoenwald SK. Evidence-based practice in child
    and adolescent mental health services. Psychiatr Serv 2001;52(9):1179–89.
[4] Torrey WC, Drake RE, Dixon L, Burns BJ, Flynn L, Rush AJ, et al. Implementing evidence-based
    practices for persons with severe mental illnesses. Psychiatr Serv 2001;52(1):45–50.
[5] Struening EL, Perlick DA, Link BG, Hellman F, Herman D, Sirey JA. Stigma as a barrier to
    recovery: the extent to which caregivers believe most people devalue consumers and their fami-
    lies. Psychiatr Serv 2001;52(12):1633–8.
[6] Tanenbaum S. Evidence-based practice in mental health: practice weaknesses meet political
    strengths. J Eval Clin Pract 2003;9(2):287–301.
[7] Birkel RC, Hall LL, Lane T, Cohan K, Miller J. Consumers and families as partners in imple-
    menting evidence-based practice. Psychiatr Clin North Am 2003;26(4):867–81.

CHILD AND
ADOLESCENT
PSYCHIATRIC CLINICS
OF NORTH AMERICA

ELSEVIER
SAUNDERS

Child Adolesc Psychiatric Clin N Am
14 (2005) 225–240

Practitioner Perspectives on Evidence-Based Practice

Mina K. Dulcan, MD[a,b,*]

[a]Child and Adolescent Psychiatry, Children's Memorial Hospital, 2300 Children's Plaza, #10, Chicago, IL 60614, USA
[b]Departments of Psychiatry and Behavioral Sciences and Pediatrics, Northwestern University, Feinberg School of Medicine, 303 East Chicago Avenue, Chicago, IL 60611, USA

Most aspiring child mental health professionals would support the premise that clinical practice should have a scientific foundation. Why, then, is the implementation of evidence-based practice (EBP) in child and adolescent psychiatry so difficult? Considering the multiple stakeholders in clinical work, impediments are not surprising. Practitioner delays in implementation of research findings are common to all specialties of medicine. This article outlines the barriers to implementation of EBP and suggests changes to motivate and enable clinicians to use EBPs.

In this article, evidence-based medicine (EBM) refers to the specific techniques (originally described in the *JAMA* series of "Users' guides to the medical literature" published between 1993 and 2000; also found in "Users' guides to the medical literature: a manual for evidence-based clinical practice. Essentials of evidence-based clinical practice [pocket version], a CD-ROM, and an interactive web site [www.usersguides.org] available from the American Medical Association) [1] of finding, appraising, and applying evidence to answer questions regarding a particular patient about which tests to use, what the results mean, and which treatment is most likely to be effective. EBP is used to mean the more general use of research to guide assessment and treatment. Other terms are used in the psychology literature, such as empirically supported treatment (EST) and empirically validated treatment (EVT), which refer to psychotherapies. Recent reviews [2–4] considered evidence-based treatments (EBTs), including psychosocial and pharmacologic interventions.

* Child and Adolescent Psychiatry, Children's Memorial Hospital, 2300 Children's Plaza, #10, Chicago, IL 60614.
  E-mail address: m-dulcan@northwestern.edu

Impediments to evidence-based practice

The evidence

Unfortunately, we do not yet have evidence that either the use of EBM in clinical decision making or the use of particular EBTs actually improves outcomes in the "real world," compared with treatment as usual.

Where is the evidence in child mental health practice? We are a relatively young field, and because of paradigm shifts in the understanding of mental problems in young people, dramatic changes in diagnostic criteria, and only recent availability of medications, the evidence base is limited. Updated compilations of evidence may be found on the Internet (eg, Centre for Evidence-Based Mental Health [http://cebmh.com/]) and in journals (eg, *Evidence-based Mental Health*, *Clinical Evidence*, and *The Scientific Review of Mental Health Practice*).

There are not enough randomized controlled trials (RCTs), and existing RCTs may not be widely applicable. Psychotherapy trials traditionally have been conducted in specialized research clinics. Industry-sponsored medication trials typically enroll highly restricted samples to maximize the cost-benefit ratio of the drug development process. There is virtually no systematic evidence on combinations of drugs and little evidence regarding combinations of psychotherapy and medication in youth (among the notable exceptions are the National Institute of Mental Health-sponsored projects: Multimodal Treatment of Attention Deficit Hyperactivity Disorder [ADHD] [MTA] and Treatment of Adolescent Depression Study [TADS]). The evidence offers little guidance on how to prioritize or combine interventions, which parts of complex treatment packages are essential, or when and how to change treatments when the patient is not improving. There are few answers to questions regarding the treatment of comorbid disorders. Selecting a particular treatment for a specific patient requires considerable extrapolation at best. Even when the results of an RCT apply, independent replications are limited for psychological and pharmacologic treatments.

The body of evidence varies with diagnosis. There are countless RCTs for ADHD, especially short-term studies of stimulants for elementary school-aged boys. In contrast, a recent review of child and adolescent eating disorders stated that "the evidence base for effective interventions is surprisingly weak" [5]. Even for extensively studied syndromes such as ADHD and anxiety disorders, there are important age gaps in the evidence. Children are different at 4, 7, 11, and 16 years of age, whereas adults from age 20 to 55 are likely to respond similarly to treatments. Rarely does the evidence even consider the spectrum of socioeconomic, ethnic, and cultural populations.

When clinicians read reports of research studies, they find that they have little in common with the persons who implement the treatment. Clinicians in research trials are most often specially trained to focus on a narrow range of disorders and techniques and seem to be treating only patients who volunteer for a particular protocol and who receive the treatment with no cost to them or involvement of third party payers.

The evidence itself is complex and often difficult to apply. In the first of the classic *JAMA* series "Users' guides to the medical literature" [6], three core questions were proposed:

1. Are the results of the study valid?
2. What are the results?
3. Will the results help me in caring for my patients?

The authors point out that the answers to these questions are rarely simple, and "evidence comes in shades of gray." The results, even of effective treatments, are rarely dramatic or universal. This also is true in the rest of medicine, because many infectious diseases are prevented or quickly treated, and management of chronic illnesses defines more of clinicians' practices. At the end of a study, the conclusion is most often not "yes" or "no," but "maybe" or "it depends." No study is perfect, and the limitations make drawing conclusions complex. As science advances, most articles in scholarly journals present bits and pieces of evidence, which may or may not subsequently be replicated. For many clinicians, a journal such as *Archives of General Psychiatry* is incomprehensible. There is an increasing gap between cutting edge research (especially in the etiology of psychiatric disorders) and the ordinary clinician.

Statistics are difficult for clinicians to interpret. For example, even a "large" effect size of 0.8 indicates that only approximately half of the treatment group had greater improvement than the average control subject. Few clinicians know (or remember) how to interpret an ANOVA or MANOVA or the increasingly complex statistical methods currently used. Statistical significance versus clinical significance may be confusing. How should a clinician interpret group mean results versus number of individuals who improve or stay the same or get worse?

There are no agreed-upon outcome measures. Different measures disagree, even those from the same informant. Discrepancies among informants are even more difficult to interpret. Most outcome measures attempt to quantify individual symptoms, not the larger family or systems issues that often are the focus of treatment. Measures of parent satisfaction do not correlate with other measures of symptomatic improvement.

There have been several prominent examples of the difficulty interpreting outcome measures. Multiple papers from the MTA study have used different analytic methods and measures in an effort to demonstrate the superiority of combined treatment. The controversy about efficacy and safety of selective serotonin reuptake inhibitors in children has been complicated by a high placebo response rate and variability among outcome measures in whether medication yields better response than placebo.

Guides to the evidence

Child and adolescent psychiatry, a young specialty among medical disciplines, has progressed from knowledge that was based almost entirely on anecdotes and expert opinions to proliferating, and perhaps confusing, resources for the clinician. An increasing number of journals, books, practice parameters, guidelines, algorithms, continuing education programs, and subscription and industry-sponsored newsletters compete for the attention of the busy practitioner. Child mental health has not been well represented in the easy-to-access Web-based compendia of clinical trials that are commonly used in internal medicine or even adult psychiatry.

The writing, approval, and implementation of practice guidelines are a work in progress. In other specialties of medicine, clinical pathways and best practices for treating disorders such as asthma or hypertension have been effective in improving outcomes and reducing cost when used in motivated settings. Although psychiatric patients are not actually more complex than other patients, we pay more attention to the complexity and may become lost in the details. Even in other specialties of medicine, however, evidence is slow to diffuse to individual practitioners in the community, and it is difficult for "experts" to agree on the details of guidelines.

An editorial commented: "As methods to protect against an ever-increasing number of lurking biases continue to improve, the clinical and scientific community may be approaching unsustainable levels of scientific purity necessary to produce and maintain the ideal evidence-based clinical guideline. Not only is the cost of current rigorous methods for producing an evidence-based guideline high, but the lag time from start to final product is severely testing the patience of those who commission and fund guideline development" [7].

Practice guidelines typically blend evidence and expert opinion, and their content and emphasis may be influenced by multiple stakeholders. If practice parameters are abbreviated and simplified to ease their use, they risk rigidity and lack of applicability to subsets of cases. Attempts to include all possible aspects and complexities result in parameters so lengthy that they are unlikely to be read and impossible to execute. Guidelines on the same topic from different sources may conflict. As the field advances, guidelines are not able to respond rapidly because of the unwieldy organizational structure that produces them. For example, the American Academy of Child and Adolescent Psychiatry (AACAP) practice parameters for the treatment of ADHD already must be modified because of the findings of the MTA, release of new formulations of stimulant medications, and the approval of an entirely new drug, atomoxetine. Conversely, guidelines that are written by one or a small group of authors, although more rapid and potentially more rigorous, risk lack of general acceptance.

Guidelines from organizations are developed by committees and risk a "guild" influence to emphasize treatments favored by their members. Because the body of evidence is insufficient, a guideline must go beyond it to be useful to clinicians. "Expert consensus" is acceptable in EBM, but it is easily distorted by special interests to include practices that clinicians prefer and believe to be effective. Industry attempts to influence guidelines (eg, whether a particular medication would be listed as first- or second-line treatment) increase suspicion when any outside funding supports the process or when the authors of guidelines have relationships with industry. Ironically, more common but covert efforts to influence treatment guidelines may stem from personal conflicts of interest, such as supporting a favored treatment method or opposing a competing one.

For patients and disorders that lack current evidence-based practice parameters, guidelines, or algorithms, clinicians must turn to chapters and review articles. These are nonsystematic and often list or summarize a mixture of clinical wisdom, historical practices, and research evidence rather than systematically and critically appraise the evidence.

Empirically supported assessment measures and treatment models

Despite progress in the past 5 years, there are still not enough empirically supported, clinically valid, and feasible evaluation and diagnostic measures and treatments. Some disorders have no EBPs at all, and others have few. Even when EBTs exist, we know little about their mechanisms of action, which parts are necessary and sufficient, and for whom and under what conditions they are most effective. We lack the evidence that ESTs can be transported from the RCT to routine practice conditions. The question of how much deviation from the original proven model is possible without losing effectiveness is largely unanswered. Even in psychopharmacology, it is not clear how strictly the clinician must adhere to the EBT package. For example, in the MTA, the best medication dose was determined by double-blind trials on a range of doses (including placebo) using daily rating scales completed by parents and teachers. Is this full procedure necessary to obtain maximal benefit from stimulant treatment? It is almost never feasible.

Even when EBPs exist, dissemination and access are limited. Many assessment measures and therapy models are proprietary, available only for sale (at a cost greater than simply reproduction and distribution) or jealously guarded against competition. For psychotherapies, even when the developers wish to disseminate them, there is no efficient or cost-effective mechanism. It often is difficult to access the manuals and materials and be trained in their use. Conversely, psychopharmacologic treatments move much more quickly into community practice. Industry rapidly disseminates information about new drugs and new indications for existing drugs. Access is as easy as a prescription pad.

Psychosocial interventions developed in a research model are difficult and expensive to implement because they require intensive instruction and ongoing close supervision to ensure fidelity. Many manual-based treatments are not compatible with a community approach to patient care. A lock-step sequence may not fit with the strengths and weaknesses or priorities of patients and families. We do not know how much flexibility may be permitted before effectiveness is lost. Clinicians trained in ESTs are not widely available in many communities, even for the simplest behavioral treatments. Some ESTs are not feasible for most office or clinic-based therapists. Multisystemic therapy (MST), for example, uses targeted family interventions and intensive and comprehensive services based in the home, school, and neighborhood.

Clinicians

Clinician barriers to EBM include attitudes and values, lack of convenient access to information resources and the skills to assimilate and appraise the available evidence, and the time required in the face of patient needs [8].

Historically, much of child mental health practice was theory based rather than evidence based. Clinicians believed that "each child is unique" and that group evidence never applied to their particular patients. We do not know the importance of each patient's unique features in determining the choice and success of treatment. Many clinicians fear that too much science drives out humanity. An unfortunate dichotomy has emerged between the art and the science of mental health practice. Those who promote the art disparage evidence from research as imperfect and therefore hopelessly flawed. They fear rigid imposition of rules for practice. "Flexibility, clinical judgment, and tailoring treatment to what therapists perceive as the unique needs of individual clients have long been considered the hallmarks of a skilled clinician." Unfortunately, in practice, narrow theoretical preferences of clinicians who do not keep up or who do not appreciate a full range of modalities may foster the application to all patients of the clinician's preferred treatment model, based on apprenticeship with powerful figures in the clinician's training. Alternatively, treatment may shift direction with every new issue or symptom presented by the patient.

Some clinicians fear loss of professional autonomy. They believe that external forces (eg, payers, certifying bodies) are imposing EBM only to save money or to exert control. Others resist sharing decision making with patients, and EBM gives authority to the data, not the physician. Practitioners may be alienated by the extreme position taken by a few evangelical proponents of EBM that disparages clinical experience and judgment.

Even the best practitioners view patients one by one and may find it difficult to "believe" the results of research: "Studies may show that drug is effective, but it hasn't worked on the first three of my patients when I tried it, so I am not going to use it any more!" Clinicians may fear that EBM will expose their current practices as obsolete and ineffective or even harmful. They fear that practice guidelines will be used as weapons in malpractice litigation.

Clinicians may dismiss EBM as demanding only the use of medication or stereotypically applied "boring" manualized therapies or "cookbook medicine" (although real cookbooks nearly always lead to better meals than random or idiosyncratic combination and heating of ingredients). They object that EBM takes the "fun" or the "art" out of clinical work. There is a common misperception that EBM rejects clinical experience and intuition and patient values and preferences, when actually these are key to the approach, along with the best available evidence from epidemiology and controlled trials.

Clinicians who seek perfect, rather than the best available, evidence may succumb to "evidence nihilism" rather than accept that all studies have flaws and limitations to generalizability [8]. Practitioners lack the tools to decide which limitations are important in application to an individual patient, whether the limitations are fatal, what is their likely effect, whether the conclusions should be rejected or tempered. In trying to use EBM, clinicians underestimate their information needs, have difficulty formulating answerable and practical questions, and become overwhelmed by the number of questions and the lists of references generated when they do searches. They do not know how to focus a search using OVID or PubMed to find the most rigorous relevant papers. They do not use EBM often enough to develop and remember the skills. A diverse practice makes keeping up with all of the evidence seem impossible. The busy clinician finds EBM too difficult and time consuming and falls back on his or her training or other sources, such as industry-sponsored talks, CME presentations at national meetings, single or review articles in journals, books, and community standards and opinion leaders. Unfortunately, in all fields of medicine, community standards are slow to change in response to research. Expert opinion often lags behind and may even be inconsistent with the evidence, especially when opinion leaders favor a particular approach.

When up-to-date synthesized guides to the evidence (eg, practice guidelines) exist, clinician barriers to adherence include lack of awareness of a guideline's existence, lack of familiarity with the specific content of the guideline, lack of agreement with the concept of guidelines or content of a specific guideline, lack of belief in ability to implement a tactic recommended by a guideline, lack of belief that implementing the guideline improves patient outcomes, and inertia of previous practice or training [9].

Clinicians find manual-based treatments mechanical or even boring to implement. They prefer flexibility, are interested in the details of people's lives, and find it easier for clinician and family to engage in unstructured conversation than to follow a prescribed sequence of interventions and homework. Community-based treatments may require therapists who are willing to go into unsavory homes and neighborhoods and be available 24/7. Few clinicians at the doctoral or even master's level wish to practice in that way.

Many clinicians are unaware that the new generation of ESTs is increasingly flexible and includes procedures for crisis intervention or "rescue." Treatment modules using various empirically supported techniques can be selected and implemented in an order tailored to the strengths, weaknesses, and preferences of the patient and family. A survey of licensed clinical psychologists (most at the PhD level) found lack of familiarity with and misconceptions about treatment manuals [10]. Some respondents believed that manualized therapies dehumanize the therapist and the client. One might expect similar beliefs among child psychiatrists, especially those not recently trained. In contrast, current well-designed treatment manuals allow considerable flexibility in implementation of prescribed interventions.

A substantial proportion of mental health clinicians are office based in fee-for-service solo private practices. Without hospital or university affiliations, they have limited access to full-text journals on-line and other resources. Realistically, EBP is more time and energy consuming than usual care. Clinicians in offices or agencies that see patients back to back, often at low managed care rates, have little time to think about EBP or implement treatments that require planning between sessions. The shortage of child and adolescent psychiatrists and the pressure of patient needs often lead child psychiatrists to limit their practice to highly focused evaluations and medication treatment.

Despite recent efforts, incorporation of EBM practices and use of EBTs into training programs is slow. Even the nature of evidence and how to evaluate it is insufficiently taught. Senior leaders and supervisors may believe that they know better and say publicly that they do not "believe in evidence-based medicine." These disparaging comments are based on a faulty and simplistic understanding of EBM and EBTs. Senior clinicians also may resist the way that EBM increases the authority of junior clinicians who are more facile with computers and the EBM method and decreases the power attributed to seniority or "in my experience." Teaching EBP requires more time and effort for trainee and faculty in an era when faculty have less time for teaching. There are insufficient supervisors with expertise in EBM or EBTs.

In many training settings, it is difficult to find "simple" patients with whom trainees can learn EBM or EBPs. Trainees select for case conferences unusual or especially challenging cases, often with multiple systems dysfunction. Discussion focuses on presumptions regarding etiology rather than implementing a structure that teaches formulation of a clinical question, search and appraisal strategies, and evaluation of how the results apply to the care of the particular patient. An EBM-format case conference requires more preparation by the trainee and more energy from faculty in the face of powerful inertia and increasing other demands on time.

Patients and families

Parents' understandable anxieties about research and the lack of attention to these concerns by investigators lead many families to be reluctant to participate in clinical trials, which makes it more difficult for the field to improve the evidence base.

A significant impediment to EBP is the lack of public understanding of the scientific method. Most Americans do not "believe" in evolution, despite overwhelming evidence! Complementary and alternative medicine therapies are increasingly popular because they are considered to be more "natural" and are therefore better. Media exposure facilitates special agendas. Some physicians give compelling testimonials to promote unproven (and highly speculative) treatments. Others with doctoral degrees use the popular media to discredit empirically supported treatments (eg, use of stimulants for ADHD). How is a parent to know whom to believe? Even well-educated parents may not understand the nature of evidence in medicine.

Understandably, parents of children with psychiatric disorders do not easily tolerate uncertainty, they want answers! The cures promised by charismatic special interest groups (or charlatans) may be more attractive than a careful weighing of the pros and cons derived from research. A particularly egregious example was the use of facilitated communication to "cure" autism. Its advocates dismissed research because facilitated communication would work only if you believe, not in a controlled trial to test it.

Families differ in their values, goals, and expectations. Some resist treatments that are clearly evidence based (eg, stimulant medication for ADHD) because they are suspicious of medications. They pay for or demand highly touted evaluations (eg, hair analysis) or treatments (eg, chiropractic manipulation) that have no evidence to support their use [11].

Assertive families want what they have heard about on television or found on the Internet. Depending on their source of information and their ability to evaluate it, this may be positive or negative. Families may feel that implementation of EBPs reduces their empowerment or choice of treatments. What is the clinician to do when a family refuses a treatment of known efficacy and insists on one that is not supported by research?

The complexity of patients makes application of EBM difficult. Because of the filters of recruitment, inclusion and exclusion criteria, and consent procedures, when compared with research subjects, community patients are likely to have more stressors and be less adherent, although recent RCTs that studied severe illnesses with recruitment from families who sought treatment (as opposed to analog studies, youth scoring high on screening measures, or rarified university psychology research clinics) have found that the lives of research subjects also are complex and stressful.

Child and adolescent psychiatrists are likely to see highly comorbid youth. There are no research data to inform the process of prioritizing the treatment of multiple diagnoses. Families present not only with comorbidity but also with an array of psychiatric and social issues: poverty, schools whose few resources are overwhelmed, dangerous neighborhoods, poor housing, and parental inability to read or even speak English. Parents of all socioeconomic groups may struggle with parental mental illness, substance abuse, marital discord, and absence of a functional parental coalition. Barriers to treatment, such as cost, transportation, and time lost from work, interfere with implementing EBTs. For example, the MTA strongly suggested the superiority of titrating initial and maintenance stimulant doses using teacher reports, but these are often difficult to obtain. Monthly medication monitoring visits seemed to be important in enhancing improvement, but in clinical settings, many parents resist monthly appointments, citing poor insurance coverage or time lost from parental work or child's school.

Unlike adult psychiatry, child mental health care is inevitably involved with parents, schools, and often other agencies, such as child protective services. So much of what we do as clinicians is not primarily about the axis I diagnosis. Sometimes parents or foster parents are unwilling or unable to expend the necessary effort. Clinicians are asked to "just fix the kid."

Institutions

Agencies serve patient populations with diverse disorders and demographics. There is a shortage of clinicians and often long waiting lists. Agencies must have sufficient clinician productivity and case loads to balance the budget. Organizational dynamics may not be amenable to implementation of ESTs. Technology and resources are limited for monitoring fidelity and assessing outcome.

Many ESTs are not feasible in a fee-for-service environment. They have been developed in research settings, often providing care for free and using trainees or staff trained and paid by research grants to provide the care.

Payers

Early in the history of managed care, there was a great deal of talk about quality indicators and outcome measures. Sadly, there has been little evidence of implementation of standards of quality, only the core motivation to deny or minimize care to assure a low "medical loss ratio" (ie, as few dollars as possible actually spent on care). Managed care and Medicaid pay for services that have no empirical support but do not pay for some ESTs, or they pay so little that they cannot be implemented.

Payer rules require that services be office or clinic based and that the therapy be applied directly to the child (a surgical model). As a result, clinics and clinicians who provide weekly individual unstructured psychotherapy for children are paid, but those who implement behavioral treatments in schools or provide empirically supported parent training are not. The requirement for the "identified patient" to be seen in order for the service to be covered leads to crowded waiting rooms, need for staff to supervise the children, and either restriction of services to after-school hours or children unnecessarily missing school.

Silos of funding for mental health services, medical care, education, child protective services, income support and housing, and juvenile justice have led to a "penny wise and pound foolish" system, in which there is insufficient funding to implement interventions that are known to be cost effective in the long run (such as Head Start and MST). In the meager funding for services for children and families, government and taxpayers do not consider the eventual expenses (not to mention human suffering) generated by poor, uneducated, mentally ill, or criminal adults.

Increasing the feasibility and implementation of evidence-based practice

How do we change the culture in favor of EBM and EBTs and speed technology transfer?

Evidence

We need more research to produce more evidence. Where RCTs have not been done or would not be feasible, N of 1 and multiple baseline or ABA trials can be used. Progress is being made studying children with comorbidity (eg, ADHD plus anxiety or disruptive behavior disorder in the MTA, stimulant treatment for children with ADHD and mental retardation). We must demonstrate that EBTs developed in research settings can be translated to the real world, improve patient outcome, and are compatible with patient and parent satisfaction. We must provide guidance in implementation. Clinicians will be motivated to invest the extra time and effort once they see published successful dissemination effectiveness trials.

We need outcome measures that reflect actual clinical improvement, not just patient or parent satisfaction, and have face validity to clinicians, with acceptable reliability and feasibility of implementation in busy practices. We need mechanisms for feedback in "real time" to clinicians of actual change in patient or family level of symptoms and adaptive functioning. We need convenient and cost-effective ways to obtain teacher ratings and observational measures, especially for children with ADHD and oppositional defiant disorder.

We must insist on statistical techniques that are relevant to clinical work and application of research results. Statistical "significance" is not enough. For evaluation measures we can use positive predictive power and negative predictive power. Useful measures for RCTs include effect size, proportion of subjects improved, normalized, or worsened, and number needed to treat (the number of patients who would need to be treated with a specified intervention to obtain one additional positive outcome or prevent one negative outcome that would not have occurred with the control condition).

Access to information and guides to the evidence

We have come a long way and have many more resources than even a few years ago. Access to PubMed via Medline is free. Organizations such as the AACAP and the American Psychiatric Association offer practice guidelines to their members. Professional organizations also could provide training in techniques of EBM and access to searchable resources.

The compendia of evidence and the empirically supported assessment measures and treatments must be readily accessible. Clinicians do not have time to search, appraise, and integrate evidence for each clinical question. They need easy-to-access, concise, integrated, and unbiased guidelines and summaries of research applied to clinical practice. There could be easily accessible and searchable banks of "critically appraised topics," frequently updated, for economy of effort.

Computer-based medical information systems can make feasible the development and use of probability-based clinical prediction rules, that is, using epidemiologic data and the known properties of tests and interventions to calculate a recommendation regarding evaluation or treatment of a specific patient. Internet searches, on-line journal access, and high-speed internet access make EBM more feasible. Making evidence quickly and easily available to clinicians has been shown to increase the extent to which evidence is sought and used [12]. The increasing number of Web-based resources with content relevant to child mental health, with their availability facilitated by bedside or handheld computers with internet access (or CD-ROMs or downloaded data bases), will facilitate this process.

Review articles, textbook chapters, and practice guidelines should systematically consider the evidence, using clear rules for literature search, evaluation of quality of studies, and summarization of findings, and make explicit the values and preferences underlying recommendations, including benefits, costs, feasibility, and preference of patients and families.

Clinical guidelines must be based on the best available evidence, not guild preferences. They must be flexible enough to allow for the values, preferences, and goals of the patient and family. The trade-offs of risk to benefit and cost to benefit should be made explicit. Factors that facilitate implementation of evidence-based family medicine guidelines in The Netherlands include a national process that takes into account feasibility in practice; process of writing that includes summaries of evidence and considerable input by clinicians and established experts; publication in a scientific journal along with the relevant scientific background information; support materials for the guideline, including plastic pocket cards and software to facilitate implementation (eg, by issuing reminders) and paper and computerized audit instruments for practitioners, summaries for receptionists, and leaflets and letters for patients; planned dissemination by regional and local continuing medical education and quality improvement coordinators; outreach visits by specially trained peer practitioners; and updating every 3 to 5 years as new evidence becomes available [13]. Additional strategies being tested include outreach by trained nurses, changes in organization of practices, and patient-mediated interventions (eg, providing guidelines directly to patients).

Practical algorithms have been developed that have data on the feasibility of their implementation in the community. Some examples (not an exhaustive list) are pharmacologic treatments of ADHD [14], depression [15], and pediatric bipolar disorder [16]. Even when the algorithms are not completely followed, their use seems to reduce polypharmacy. Parental satisfaction is not hindered. Computerized "real time" reminder systems could facilitate clinician adherence to the monitoring recommendations in practice guidelines.

Implementation of EBPs must be convenient for busy clinicians and trainees. If the collection and appraisal of evidence have been done for a particular disorder, an "auditable protocol" can be created to standardize agreed-upon minimal elements of care that can be checked off by the clinician for self-monitoring (or by others for quality assurance) [17]. The Columbia Treatment Guidelines Project (David Shaffer, MD, and Jami Young, PhD, personal communication, 2003) provides printed guidelines with copies of assessment instruments, instructions for implementation of particular techniques, and handouts for parents.

Measures and models

Typically, treatment manuals are designed to assure internal validity in an RCT. We need a new generation of modularized ESTs that are meant for implementation in the community with that research data on which deviations from protocol are permissible and are likely to lead to ineffective treatment. If ESTs are to be feasible and effective in clinical practice, they must be designed and tested with the "messiness" of the real world in mind, with the populations, clinicians, and clinical settings that resemble usual care in the community.

EBPs must be disseminated to be used. All journals could adopt a policy (as the *Journal of the American Academy of Child and Adolescent Psychiatry* has done) that requires that unpublished assessment measures and treatment manuals be made available, either on request from the author (free or for the cost of copying and shipping) or linked to the journal on-line. Funding agencies could mandate and support dissemination of valid measures and effective interventions. Personal profit (beyond the expenses to produce materials and time in teaching and supervision) from the fruits of taxpayer-funded research should be discouraged.

Rotheram-Borus and Duan [18] suggested a private enterprise model for development and dissemination of preventive interventions that could apply equally well to treatment interventions. Others have suggested that dissemination efforts be modeled on those used by pharmaceutical companies, which often lead to surprisingly rapid clinician behavior change in the frequency of prescribing a drug. Some ESTs already have been packaged for easy dissemination (eg, Webster-Stratton's video-based parent training program, the Incredible Years Series), and more could follow.

Clinicians

There is hope for the newer generations, trained under the requirements of accrediting bodies for inclusion of EBP in psychiatric residencies and use of ESTs in psychology training programs. New residents and practicing psychiatrists have learned to use EBM methods in medical school. Graduate schools of social work are beginning to adopt EBPs.

Students and practicing clinicians must learn to use electronic databases to define problems and search for evidence, ask focused questions, critically appraise the validity and quality of the evidence and the applicability of the research results to a particular clinical situation, and determine which type of evidence is most appropriate. Although systematic review or an RCT might be best for a question about treatment effectiveness, for other questions, qualitative approaches, case-control studies, and population surveys are more appropriate [8]. EBM strategies can be offered as continuing education and in professional society-sponsored journals.

Innovative ways are needed to train practitioners in ESTs in child mental health. Surgeons visit each other to learn new procedures, but the time course of therapy prohibits this. New technology could be used in initial learning of new models and ongoing supervision.

Given the lack of evidence that conventional educational strategies influence practitioners in the direction of EBP, various tactics have been suggested, including interactive educational sessions, academic detailing or outreach visits to practice settings, manual or computerized reminders to perform a clinical inter-vention, audit of practice with feedback, efforts by opinion leaders (respected expert peers) to influence practice patterns, contacts with patients by other individuals to provide education or counseling or to collect information that is then turned over to the provider, and social marketing, in which specific barriers to change are identified and targeted [19].

Hamilton [20] suggested that "evidence-based thinking" can be used to improve the therapeutic alliance by teaching parents and adolescents how to think about the evidence and choose among or prioritize treatments, sort fact from opinion, encourage shared decision making, and foster realistic expectations of treatment. The "art" of child psychiatric practice is preserved in developing an understanding of the child's disorder and its context, communicating that understanding and the relevant evidence to the patient and family, listening to the response, and developing a therapeutic alliance in which the "science" and family values and preferences can be considered and the best available evidence applied to the particular clinical situation. What is being eliminated is the clinician's personal or theoretical preferences for treatment modalities. Parents arrive with ideas gleaned from direct-to-consumer advertising or the Internet; EBM can help clinicians and parents sort truth from fiction.

While awaiting more and better evidence, Nock et al [21] suggested an approach to psychotherapy treatment similar to that used in psychopharmacology, in which "off label" prescription is common, based on child, parent, and family factors. The premise is that treatment that is partially empirically supported is better than treatment with no empirical support at all, as long as each case is approached using systematic data collection and evaluation of effectiveness. We must foster the view in clinicians that each case is an N of 1 study, with as empirical an approach as possible to evaluation, selection of interventions, and ongoing assessment of progress.

Patients and families

Computer technology awaits only funding and effort to develop interactive guides (Web-based or CD-ROM) for patients and families that provide custom-ized information about disorders and therapeutic alternatives to enhance and make more feasible shared decision making.

Institutions

A useful example from adult psychiatry is the Implementing Evidence-Based Practices for Severe Mental Illness Project to promote the use of specific EBPs in the public sector. The project has developed tool kits that contain written materials, didactic and experiential training opportunities, Web-based resources, and ongoing supervision and consultation. Tool kits are developed not only for clinicians but also for payers, administrators, consumers, and family members. The three core strategies are packaging the EBPs to make them easy to use, teaching and motivating providers to use them, and shaping the organizational context in which they are to be used [22].

A more radical suggestion is to create a cadre of master's- or even bachelor's-level therapists trained in particular models of ESTs that is supervised by doctoral-level clinicians who have the depth and breadth of education and experience necessary to perform comprehensive assessment and design and monitor treatment plans. One model is MST, which recruits motivated, bright, and energetic master's-level therapists, trains them specifically, and supervises them closely for treatment adherence and creative problem solving regarding barriers to treatment progress. Therapists are taught the ESTs rather than the process of EBM.

Payers

We desperately need increased funding and integration of the entire spectrum of educational and social services for children and families. There must be a financial incentive structure to encourage EBP and discourage the use of nonspecific or unproven therapies that waste time, money, and precious clinical resources. Providers could be rewarded for outcomes or, until that technology is improved, at least for the use of best practices and incorporation of evaluation measures rather than for hours of service rendered.

Summary

Various barriers impede the use of EBM and the implementation of empirically supported assessment measures and treatments. Progress is being made, and tactics are proposed to motivate clinicians and speed the transfer of research findings to community practice.

References

[1] Gray GE. Concise guide to evidence-based psychiatry. Washington, DC: American Psychiatric Publishing; 2004.
[2] McClellan JM, Werry JS. Evidence-based treatments in child and adolescent psychiatry: an inventory. J Am Acad Child Adolesc Psychiatry 2003;42(12):1388–400.
[3] Kazdin AE, Weisz JR, editors. Evidence-based psychotherapies for children and adolescents. New York: Guilford Press; 2003.
[4] Lilienfeld SO, Lynn SJ, Lohr JM, editors. Science and pseudoscience in clinical psychology. New York: Guilford Press; 2003.
[5] Gowers S, Bryant-Waugh R. Management of child and adolescent eating disorders: the current evidence base and future directions. J Child Psychol Psychiatry 2004;45(1):63–83.
[6] Oxman AD, Sackett DL, Guyatt GH. Users' guides to the medical literature. I. How to get started. JAMA 1993;270(17):2093–5.
[7] Browman GP. Development and aftercare of clinical guidelines: the balance between rigor and pragmatism. JAMA 2001;286(12):1509–11.
[8] Ramchandani P, Joughin C, Zwi M. Evidence-based child and adolescent mental health services: oxymoron or brave new dawn? Child Psychol Psychiatry Rev 2001;6(2):59–64.

[9] Cabana MD, Rushton JL, Rush AJ. Implementing practice guidelines for depression: applying a new framework to an old problem. Gen Hosp Psychiatry 2002;24(1):35–42.

[10] Addis ME, Krasnow AD. A national survey of practicing psychologists' attitudes toward psychotherapy treatment manuals. J Consult Clin Psychol 2000;68(2):331–9.

[11] Chan E. The role of complementary and alternative medicine in attention-deficit hyperactivity disorder. Dev Behav Pediatr 2002;23(1S):S37–45.

[12] Sackett DL, Straus SE. Finding and applying evidence during clinical rounds: the evidence cart. JAMA 1998;280(15):1336–8.

[13] Grol R. Successes and failures in the implementation of evidence-based guidelines for clinical practice. Med Care 2001;39(Suppl 2):II-46–54.

[14] Pliszka SR, Lopez M, Crismon ML, Toprac MG, Hughes CW, Emslie GJ, et al. A feasibility study of the Children's Medication Algorithm Project (CMAP) algorithm for the treatment of ADHD. J Am Acad Child Adolesc Psychiatry 2003;42(3):279–87.

[15] Emslie GJ, Hughes CW, Crismon ML, Lopez M, Pliszka S, Toprac MG, et al. A feasibility study of the Childhood Depression Medication Algorithm: the Texas Children's Medication Algorithm Project (CMAP). J Am Acad Child Adolesc Psychiatry 2004;43:519–27.

[16] Pavuluri MN, Henry DB, Devineni B, Carbray JA, Naylor MW, Janicak PG. A pharmacotherapy algorithm for stabilization and maintenance of pediatric bipolar disorder. J Am Acad Child Adolesc Psychiatry 2004;43:859–67.

[17] Hill P, Taylor E. An auditable protocol for treating attention deficit/hyperactivity disorder. Arch Dis Child 2001;84(5):404–9.

[18] Rotheram-Borus MJ, Duan N. Next generation of preventive interventions. J Am Acad Child Adolesc Psychiatry 2003;42(5):518–26.

[19] Hoge MA, Tondora J, Stuart GW. Training in evidence-based practice. Psychiatr Clin North Am 2003;26(4):851–65.

[20] Hamilton JD. Evidence-based thinking and the alliance with parents. J Am Acad Child Adolesc Psychiatry 2004;43(1):105–8.

[21] Nock MK, Goldman JL, Wang Y, Albano AM. From science to practice: the flexible use of evidence-based treatment in clinical settings. J Am Acad Child Adolesc Psychiatry 2004;43: 777–80.

[22] Corrigan PW, Steiner L, McCracken SG, Blaser B, Barr M. Strategies for disseminating evidence-based practices to staff who treat people with serious mental illness. Psychiatr Serv 2001; 52(12):1598–606.

ELSEVIER
SAUNDERS

Child Adolesc Psychiatric Clin N Am
14 (2005) 241–254

CHILD AND
ADOLESCENT
PSYCHIATRIC CLINICS
OF NORTH AMERICA

Theories Related to Changing Clinician Practice

Manuel Riemer, MS[a],*, Julie Rosof-Williams, RN, MSN[a,b],
Leonard Bickman, PhD[a,c]

[a]Department of Psychology and Human Development, Vanderbilt University, 1818 South Ave Drive,
Nashville, TN 37203, USA
[b]Department of Pediatrics, Vanderbilt University School of Medicine,
21st Avenue South at Garland Avenue, Nashville, TN 37232, USA
[c]Center for Evaluation and Program Improvement, Peabody College, 1212 21st Avenue South,
Nashville, TN 37203, USA

Extensive effort and resources have been dedicated to improving mental health services for children and adolescents since Jane Knitzer's report, "Unclaimed Children" stimulated the field in the early 1980s [1]. Recent approaches to reforming mental health services primarily have focused on the system level, such as the System of Care and wraparound movements, or on the treatment level, such as the promotion of evidence-based practice. The success of these system-wide and treatment-level approaches, however, ultimately is dependent on the clinicians who work within these systems and provide the treatments. If frontline clinicians do not embrace these reforms and make appropriate changes to their clinical practice, then an improvement in children's mental health outcomes cannot be expected. In this article, the authors (1) discuss factors relevant to the internal change processes that clinicians face in the adoption and implementation of evidence-based treatments (EBTs); (2) present a theory about the cognitive-affective processes that affect clinicians' motivation to change; and (3) discuss how these processes at the microlevel relate to other, more macrolevel theories of clinician practice change.

The importance of taking clinician behavior into account

EBTs in the mental health field have been defined "as clearly specified psychological treatments shown to be efficacious in controlled research with a

* Corresponding author. Center for Evaluation and Program Improvement, Peabody College, 1212 21st Avenue South, Nashville, TN 37203.

E-mail address: manuel.riemer@vanderbilt.edu (M. Riemer).

1056-4993/05/$ – see front matter © 2005 Elsevier Inc. All rights reserved.
doi:10.1016/j.chc.2004.05.002
childpsych.theclinics.com

delineated population" [2]. Included in this definition are medical and school-based interventions as they have been discussed in articles found elsewhere in this special journal issue. As the other contributions in this issue have demonstrated, many EBTs are available today; however, the literature that documents the EBTs that are used in practice shows that most clinicians do not use EBTs in their routine practice of treating clients [2–5]. Not fully implementing EBTs in everyday practice also applies to medicine, which has produced ever-increasing numbers of practice guidelines and parameters but has been troubled by low levels of adoption among clinicians [6]. This discrepancy suggests that the development and publication of EBTs do not easily lead to their increased use in practice. Among other factors (eg, the transportability of the treatment from university laboratory into clinical practice), the faithful and full adoption and implementation of EBTs can require significant behavioral change from clinicians, and such change is a complex process.

Practice change is related to many factors including characteristics of the EBT, the clients, the service delivery, the organization, and the service system [7]. There is a need to study all of the factors affecting adoption and implementation of EBTs because "the fact remains that progression from effective treatments to their implementation and dissemination in real world clinical practice settings is through largely uncharted scientific territory" [8]. This article, however, focuses attention on the cognitive-affective processes involved in the clinician behavior change process in adopting EBTs because applied theories of clinicians' cognitive-affective processes are rare and may prove to be powerful explanatory devices. Before these microlevel processes of clinician behavior change are described in more detail, some of the more macrolevel processes that individuals experience when adopting an EBT are considered. This consideration will facilitate the understanding of the function of the microprocesses in the larger context of change.

Macrolevel processes of adopting an evidence-based treatment

Everett Rogers' text *Diffusion of Innovations* [9] outlines some of the more macrolevel change processes from the perspective of individuals who have the power to adopt or reject new innovations, such as a specific EBT. According to Rogers [9], change process starts when clinicians become aware of a new EBT and gain understanding of how the EBT could be applied in the clinical setting. Clinicians become aware of new EBTs by active or passive means. If actively seeking information, clinicians may speak with peers, explore the professional literature, and thus become motivated to discover more about an EBT. If awareness occurs passively, external sources may have been involved and the clinician may have little interest or motivation in learning about the EBT. Whether awareness occurs actively or passively, clinicians may experience a "need" to explore the options for personal use of the EBT if they perceive that the EBT improves a deficit (ie, the current treatment is seen as less than efficacious). Rogers [9] explains a need as "...a state of dissatisfaction or frustration that occurs when an individual's desires outweigh the individual's actualities" (p. 172).

Typically, in Roger's thinking, when clinicians choose (active) or are required (passive) to learn more about an EBT, they will form a favorable or unfavorable attitude toward the EBT. This part of the process involves the clinician making a judgment about the credibility of the EBT's creator or sponsors. Clinicians weigh the relative advantage of the EBT against their current clinical practice, examine the compatibility of the new EBT with current clinical practices, identify clinical infrastructures available to support the new EBT, and identify the complexity of the new EBT. If the advantages outweigh the disadvantages, then the clinician engages in experimental activities that may lead to the adoption or rejection of the new EBT. During this stage, clinicians may try out the new EBT with a small sample of clients or implement part of the EBT recommendations to see how they work. If the clinician decides to fully adopt the EBT, then it will be integrated into the clinical practice. During this stage, the clinician may have altered the implementation of the EBT for a variety of reasons that include but are not limited to the clinical setting, client population, resources, or lack of understanding of the procedure or theoretic basis of the EBT. Measuring implementation fidelity and providing the clinicians with implementation fidelity feedback is a method to maintain motivation to implement the practice with fidelity [10]. Finally, the clinician who adopts the EBT will seek out feedback or confirmation that the decision to adopt the EBT was a valid and worthwhile endeavor. During this stage, clinicians decide whether they want to continue to use the EBT.

Clinicians change their practice of and beliefs about treatments for several reasons. Change that affects professional development can result from maturation or from the repetition associated with a familiar task or skill. Although these are important changes, this article focuses on the type of change that is purposeful and involves thoughtful examination of current clinical practices, professional goals, and an individual's ability to implement new clinical practices involved in using EBTs. In addition, the authors believe that clinicians ultimately control the quality and quantity of any EBT implementation for the clients they treat. Given this control, it is paramount to consider the motivation and ability of clinicians to change at the microlevel.

Microlevel processes of clinician change: motivation and ability

Motivation

Motivation often is described as intrinsic or extrinsic in nature. According to Green (as quoted in Fox et al [11]) "intrinsic motivation comes from within the individual and is comprised of urges, wishes, feelings, emotions, desires, and drives. Extrinsic motivation comes from outside the individual and is manifest in those environmental factors that precipitate behavior" (p. 18). Clinicians, like most other professionals, see their behavior and learning as self-determined [11,12]. Consequently, motivational strategies based on external pressure may have short-lived effects and run the risk of generating resentment and resistance. In many cases, the initiator for adopting new EBTs is not necessarily the clinicians, but rather the organizational leadership. That is, the process of becoming aware of the EBT is passive and, therefore, internal motivation to adopt and implement the EBT might be low. Since the direct beneficiaries of practice change most often are the clients (through more effective treatment) and, in some cases, the organization (through more efficient and cost-effective services) the clinician may not directly benefit from a practice change and thus may not have a strong motivation to change. Consequently, implementation of an EBT requires special attention to those factors that motivate change.

Ability

Motivation is a necessary but not sufficient condition for behavior change. Ability—the knowledge, clinical skills, and innate talents clinicians currently hold or obtain through additional training or learning—encompasses another set of critical factors. Clinicians' knowledge includes the understanding of disease processes, treatment regimens, current practices, and deficits in clinical practices, and recognition of discrepancies between current and desired practices. Skills are the practical clinical methods that clinicians employ to address clients' needs, and talent is the innate ability to apply specific knowledge and skills in a competent and even artful manner.

Learning is the most common activity assumed to affect clinicians' ability. As adult learners, clinicians are best served by educational interventions that involve them in the development and implementation of the educational program [13]. Empiric evidence indicates that clinicians can improve their clinical knowledge and skills [14,15]. As stated earlier, however, clinicians en mass are not adopting EBT recommendations. Thus, it appears that learning, like motivation, is a necessary but also insufficient prerequisite to the adoption of new EBTs.

In addition to internal clinician factors (ie, motivation and ability), factors external to the clinician also influence the adoption of EBTs. For example, the organization in which clinicians work (ie, organizational climate [16]), their supervisors (ie, level of support), their professional society (ie, professional norms), their peers (ie, attitudes toward EBTs), and their clients (ie, demand for the most effective and EBTs) influence the behavior of clinicians. Although the authors do not discuss these factors in detail here, their general effects on the motivation of clinicians are considered. The perceived level of support, for example, is considered as it affects the clinicians' goal expectation.

To summarize, EBTs, although established and recognized by professional associations, are not being used in routine clinical practice. Although external factors can facilitate or impede clinician change, the focus of this article is on the cognitive-affective processes believed necessary for clinician motivation to change. The two major internal clinician factors involved in the change process are motivation and ability.

Cognitive-affective processes for motivation to change

To better understand clinicians' motivation to change, the authors explored, analyzed, and synthesized current theories, scientific evidence, and expert opinions about the cognitive-affective processes involved in the purposeful changes that clinicians make in their professional practice. More specifically, Riemer and Bickman [17,18] (1) evaluated the literature for relevant research findings and theories, (2) identified the most important constructs, (3) synthesized the constructs into one coherent model, and (4) translated this model into an applied theory of guided behavior change, which they called the "Contextualized Feedback Intervention Theory" (CFIT). In the following sections, the authors apply the CFIT to clinician behavior change in the context of adopting and implementing EBTs.

Many theories of behavior change identify a perceived discrepancy between a desired goal state and the actual, current state as the key motivational force for change [11,19–23]. For example, a clinician who is committed to provide the best care possible might realize that current clinical practices are not effective. This discrepancy motivates the clinician to seek out new, more effective treatments or to implement current treatments more effectively. Given this process and its complexity, the authors draw on a range of theoretic constructs including goal commitment theory, feedback theories, cognitive dissonance theory, and causal attribution theory to describe the internal cognitive-affective processes of clinicians.

Based on the synthesis of these theories, the process of guiding a clinician to make a behavior change may follow a predetermined path. Fig. 1 provides an overview of this hypothesized path. Clinicians have to (1) be committed to the target goal (ie, implementing an EBT); (2) recognize when they have not accomplished this goal; (3) be motivated to move toward the goal; and (4) be ready to accept personal responsibility if they are not moving toward the goal.

Goal commitment is defined as "the determination to try for a goal and the persistence in pursuing it over time" [24]. Goal commitment mainly is influenced by two factors: goal attractiveness and goal expectancy [24,25]. Goal attractiveness is the subjective valence that a certain goal has for the individual. This valence is based on the perceived instrumentality that the goal has for other higher order goals [26]. The goal of implementing an EBT can be attractive because it is perceived as improving the effectiveness of current practice (active) or because non-EBTs will not be reimbursed by the insurance company (passive/reactive). Goal expectancy—the belief in the ability to accomplish the goal—is formed through an assessment of one's own capabilities (self-efficacy) and supportive factors and barriers in the form of competing goals and activities in accomplishing the goal [25,27–29].

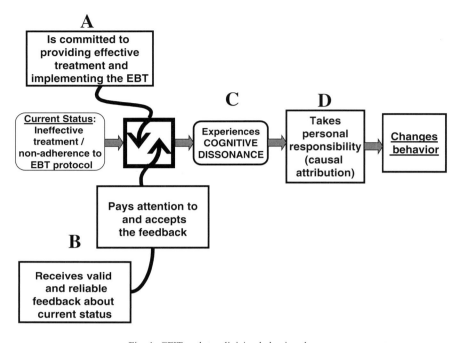

Fig. 1. CFIT path to clinician behavior change.

Examples of barriers to the implementation of an EBT might be time constraints, excessive paperwork, or lack of reimbursement for certain activities, whereas supportive factors could be resources for training and extensive supervision, among others. The issue of barriers has been described and studied more extensively in the context of competing demands models [30,31]. Real-world service settings are complex and influenced by many factors including regulatory concerns, contracts, leadership and supervision, and organizational climate [32–34]. Understanding whether clinicians in an organization feel competent to implement a new EBT and determining which barriers they perceive as most problematic are important factors in considering interventions to increase goal commitment.

To be motivated to change, the clinician must not only be committed to the target goal but also believe that the goal is yet to be accomplished. For example, if the goal is to provide more effective services by implementing a new EBT, the clinicians must believe that the service currently being providing is not sufficiently effective. Important for self-regulated motivation to change is a feedback cue that indicates the discrepancy between the current status (ie, current behavior or practice) and a standard to be accomplished (goal) [19–23]. Because most available feedback cues in clinical practice are not systematic and reliable, clinicians frequently do not have an accurate perception of their own performance and, therefore, are likely to settle at a lower level of performance prematurely. Thus, providing systematic external feedback (eg, scores from clinical outcome measures) can be effective by launching a motivational self-regulatory mechanism of change [35,36].

The method of providing systematic outcome-based feedback about clients to clinicians evolved in the context of patient-focused psychotherapy research as a promising approach to improving client outcomes through affecting clinician behavior [36–38]. In the authors' model, the effectiveness of feedback is influenced, in part, by the level of attention that the clinician pays to the feedback and the degree to which he or she accepts the feedback as accurate (acceptance) [17]. The clinician's level of attention given to the feedback is influenced by the perceived validity and utility of the feedback, the availability and importance of competing feedback cues, and the individual's general feedback propensity.

Attention to the feedback

In planning a feedback intervention, attention should be given to the issue of perceived validity and utility because it offers the best leverage point for improving the effectiveness of external feedback. More specifically, the perceived credibility of the feedback source and the information value strongly influence the assessment of validity and utility and, thus, the level of attention paid to the feedback [39]. Another influence on perceived validity and utility is the form of the feedback. Feedback can be idiosyncratic or it can be compared with a norm or a benchmark. It can be neutral or contain an evaluative judgment. It can be delivered verbally, in writing, in graphic form, in person, or by way of a computer. Choosing these options should be based on the context of the organization where the feedback will be provided. Feedback also can differ in its complexity, although it has been suggested that feedback should be as cognitively simple as possible [40,41]. Another important aspect of the feedback is whether it simply provides information about the outcomes of one's performance (knowledge of results) or whether it is instructive or formative [42]. Feedback that also includes suggestions for improvement often is more effective in improving performance than simply providing knowledge of results. Feedback is best provided in a timely manner.

Acceptance of the feedback

Although it is important to consider these different aspects of feedback to increase attention, taking them into account does not guarantee that clinicians will use the feedback to evaluate their own performance. If the feedback message differs too greatly from their own perception of their behavior, then they are likely to reject it without further consideration. This is a likely occurrence if the feedback is negative. To preserve their self-concept, people are more likely to seek out and accept feedback information that is aligned with their positive self-image [43,44]. This self-serving bias can be viewed as a consequence of the desire to avoid dissonance-arousing information [43,45,46]. To prevent this from occurring, it is important to create a safe environment in which the clinicians do not believe that their overall self-image as a professional is threatened by the feedback but instead can accept the feedback as a way to become an even better and more effective clinician. One way to do this is to focus on the ineffectiveness of the current treatment rather than on the clinician.

If the commitment to the target goal (eg, providing effective care) is paired with the realization that the current behavior is not consistent with that goal (eg, no significant improvement in clinical outcomes over the course of treatment), then the person is likely to experience cognitive dissonance. Cognitive dissonance occurs when two personally relevant cognitions are dissonant, that is, they logically contradict each other. This contradiction creates a state of arousal, which is psychologically uncomfortable and motivates the person to reduce dissonance [45,47,48]. This dissonance constitutes one leverage point through which a motive for behavior change can be created. The CFIT takes advantage of this leverage point. Although previous theories, especially self-regulation, control, and goal-setting theories, also have described a discrepancy between a goal standard and performance as a motivational force for behavior change [19–23,49], they have not included cognitive dissonance as a possible mediator. Although cognitive dissonance can be considered only a hypothetic construct, it has great value for providing an explanation of why a realized goal-behavior discrepancy does not necessarily lead to behavior change.

According to dissonance theory, individuals have several ways to reduce dissonance (changing behavior is only one way). Dissonance can be reduced by altering the commitment to the goal (providing effective care), by making discrepant behavior less relevant, [45,48], or by attributing a failure to provide effective services to external factors. For clinicians to engage in behavior change as a consequence of a perceived discrepancy, they must remain committed to the target goal, accept that they have some personal responsibility for the failure to meet the target goal, and believe that they have some control over the factors that caused the failure [50]. In the context of implementing an EBT, it is important that the clinician makes some internal and somewhat stable causal attribution to be motivated to engage in the learning that is necessary for implementing a new treatment. If the clinician believes that the problem is simply a lack of effort, then the most likely response is to increase effort. Thus, for clinicians to be motivated to change the way treatment is done they have to attribute the problem at least partially to the current type of treatment. Demonstrating to clinicians that providing effective care is feasible by implementing EBTs and supporting them by providing tools, training, and supervision might improve clinicians' feeling of control over and responsibility for providing more effective services.

To summarize, it has been demonstrated that behavior change is not a simple process but instead involves several psychologic factors that need to come together for clinicians to change their behavior to adopt and implement an EBT. External feedback is a useful intervention to instigate self-regulated behavior change because it provides the clinicians with information on whether they are accomplishing the goal of providing effective treatment. This intervention, however, will work only if they are committed to this goal. If providing effective care is a personal goal of the clinician, then this will serve well as the higher-level goal for implementing an EBT. It is critical that the clinicians' belief that the current treatment is not sufficiently effective and that implementing the selected EBT will improve effectiveness to a degree higher than any other kind of behavior change. If, however, providing the most effective care for a client is not an important personal goal for the clinician, then another higher-level goal must be substituted, such as financial incentives or pressure from the supervisor.

It should be clear from the previous discussion that information about clinician factors is crucial in planning a successful implementation of an EBT in an organization. Before implementing an EBT there should be an assessment of possible problems (readiness assessment). Moreover, the implementation should be monitored as these factors are dynamic and will likely change over time. Riemer and Bickman have developed a battery of instruments that can be used for both readiness assessments and monitoring. These instruments are available from the authors on request. Based on the assessment with these instruments, a problem diagnostic can be accomplished and the appropriate targeted interventions can be planned.

It will not always be necessary to implement a new EBT to make current practice more effective. Sometimes it might be sufficient to increase effort, shift attention, or make other, smaller changes such as learning more about a certain diagnostic procedure. The authors' model also applies in these situations because for self-directed behavior change to occur, goal commitment, awareness that something needs to be changed, and the right causal attribution (eg, lack of effort) also are required. For example, Bickman and Riemer currently are applying the CFIT in several studies in which they are trying to affect clinicians' attention to the therapeutic working relationship with their clients and their caregivers by providing the clinicians with client-based therapeutic alliance feedback.

How the authors' model relates to other applied theories of clinician practice change

The cognitive-affective process for motivation to change is just one microlevel aspect of the practice change process. It is useful to consider how the authors' affective-cognitive model is related to other applied models and theories of practice change because the common processes could identify possibilities to simultaneously intervene at the micro- and macrolevels to produce the most effective change.

In some respects, the authors' model is similar to Prochaska's and his colleague's transtheoretic model of change [51–53], in that they both stress the importance of understanding the psychologic state of the individual and recommend individualizing interventions. These researchers state that these are five stages of change that range from people who show no motivation at all (pre-contemplation) to people who have been active in change for more than 6 months (maintenance). Prochaska and colleagues suggest that a change in the relative ratio of perceived pros (strong principle of progress) and cons (weak principle of progress) for behavior change predicts a shift in the individual's stage of change [54]. This ratio of pros and cons, however, may not do justice to the complex change processes described previously. For example, the authors believe that consideration must be given to how a change in pros or cons influences goal attractiveness (ie, clinician wants to achieve goal) and goal expectancy (ie, clinician believes the standard can be met). In addition, Bandura [55] persuasively argued that stages of change are not true stages, but rather artificial constructs, and the time cutoff points for different stages are arbitrary. The authors' approach attempts to describe behavior change as an ongoing process and recognizes the dynamic nature of change.

Additional prerequisites for EBT implementation, including clinician awareness of EBT and individual clinician characteristics, are addressed by Rogers [9], who defines diffusion as "the process in which an innovation is communicated through certain channels over time among the members of a social system" (p. 5). Communication processes (eg, discussion with colleagues, continuing education events, mass media campaigns) are leverage points for interventions. Additional evidence suggests that the characteristics of earlier adopters and later adopters differ significantly [9]. More specifically, earlier adopters are characterized by increased communication with groups internal and external to their community, increased control of financial resources, increased understanding of new technologies, and more tolerance of the uncertainties associated with the implementation of new innovations such as EBTs. Earlier adopters often are sought by change agents to assist in the spread of an innovation because they help to decrease the uncertainty that later adopters perceive as a barrier to accepting new innovations. The authors' theory delineates further the more microlevel and internal processes for adoption of EBTs and identifies additional leverage points for interventions. For example, it might be helpful for targeting an intervention to determine whether late adopters are hesitant because the goal of implementing an EBT is unattractive to them or because their goal expectancy is low.

The authors stress in their model the need to diagnose individual clinician influences before an EBT is implemented and to monitor cognitive-affective processes during the implementation process. Green and Kreuter [56] suggest a similar procedure in their precede–proceed model of health promotion planning. Predisposing factors (eg, motivating factors) influence the goal attractiveness of adopting and implementing an EBT and, to a certain degree, the goal expectancy (especially self-efficacy). Enabling factors facilitate or hinder an individual's ability to implement change. They include new skills needed to implement the EBT; availability and accessibility of resources; and laws, priorities, and commitment to change in the organization and government. Enabling factors are similar to what have been described earlier as barriers and supportive factors and, thus, influence goal expectancy, which in turn affects goal commitment. This view is aligned with the authors' argument that there are two motivational processes: motivation to adopt the EBT and motivation to implement it with fidelity over time. To reinforce adoption of EBTs, the authors have suggested that EBT implementation should be accompanied by implementation fidelity feedback. The CFIT instrumentation has been designed to help with the planning of feedback interventions for adoption and implementation and, thus, might a good supplementary tool for diagnosing issues related to reinforcing factors (see Bickman et al [10]).

Finally, the authors' approach should be combined with interventions developed in the field of adult learning theory and continuing medical education. As explained earlier, motivation is just one aspect of behavior change. Another important aspect is increase in ability, which is learning. Thus, this approach could be used to create motivation to learn about a certain EBT, and adult-learning strategies could be used effectively to facilitate a clinician's learning of the knowledge and skills needed to implement the EBT.

Summary

Implementing EBTs is a difficult endeavor that often requires clinicians to significantly change their practice behavior. This article has illustrated how changing clinician behavior is a complex process that involves clinicians' motivation and ability, while recognizing additional factors external to the clinician that might hinder or enhance adoption of EBTs. No one intervention or solution will fit all clinicians and EBT adoption situations. As stated by Oxman and colleagues [57], there are no "magic bullets." Planning the implementation of EBT requires respecting the uniqueness of individual clinicians and the development of targeted and tailored interventions. The policy implications of this model are significant. If the theory is correct, then a great deal of thought and resources need to be devoted to the implementation and long term adoption of EBTs and other clinician activities. Simply providing technical training or support, especially those that consist of a single workshop, will not be an effective way to effect change. Major change activities will require careful planning and sequencing of activities that recognize the complexity of the change process. While this process will take resources and slow down the introduction of EBTs, the authors believe that in the long run we will all benefit from more widely adopted EBTs that retain their fidelity.

Acknowledgments

The authors gratefully acknowledge Lynne Wighton's comments and editing efforts.

References

[1] Knitzer J. Unclaimed children. Washington, DC: Children's Defense Fund; 1982.
[2] Hollon S, Thase M, Markowitz J. Treatment and prevention of depression. Psychol Sci 2002;
    3(2):39–77.
[3] Beutler LE. David and Goliath: when empirical and clinical standards of practice meet. Am
    Psychol 2000;55(9):997–1007.
[4] Gonzales J, Ringeisen H, Chambers D. The tangled and thorny path of science to practice:
    tensions in interpreting and applying "evidence. Clin Psychol-Sci Pr 2002;9(2):204–9.
[5] Plante T, Boccaccini M, Andersen E. Attitudes concerning professional issues impacting psy-
    chotherapy practice among members of the American Board of Professional Psychology. Psy-
    chother-Theor Res 1998;35(1):34–42.
[6] Cabana MD, Rand CS, Rowe NR, Wu AW, Wilson MH, Abboud PC, et al. Why don't physi-
    cians follow clinical practice guidelines. JAMA 1999;282(15):1458–65.
[7] Schoenwald SK, Hoagwood K. Effectiveness, transportability, and dissemination of interven-
    tions: what matters when? Psychiatr Serv 2001;52(9):1190–7.
[8] Hoagwood K. Making the transition from research to its application: the Je Ne Sais Pas of
    evidence-based practices. Clin Psychol-Sci Pr 2002;9(2):210–3.
[9] Rogers EM. Diffusion of innovations. 5th edition. New York: Free Press; 2003.
[10] Mulvaney S, Riemer M, Bickman L. How to design and implement a contextualized feedback
    intervention. Issues in design and measurement. Presented at the 16th Annual Research Con-
    ference, A System of Care for Children's Mental Health: Expanding the Research Base. Tampa,
    FL; 2003.
[11] Fox RD, Mazmanian PE, Putnam RW. Changing and learning in the lives of physicians. New
    York: Praeger; 1989.
[12] Cantillon P, Jones R. Does continuous medical education in general practice make a difference?
    BMJ 1999;318:1276–9.
[13] Knowles M. The adult learner: a neglected species. 4th edition. Houston (TX): Gulf Publishing
    Co.; 1990.
[14] Davis DA, Thomson O'Brien MA, Oxman AD, Haynes RB. Evidence for the effectiveness of
    CME. A review of 50 randomized controlled trials. JAMA 1992;268(9):1111–7.
[15] Davis D. Does CME work? An analysis of the effect of educational activities on physician
    performance or health care outcomes. Int J Psychiat Med 1998;28(1):21–39.
[16] Glisson C, Hemmelgarn A. The effects of organizational climate and interorganizational coor-
    dination on the quality and outcomes of children's service systems. Child Abuse Negl 1998;
    22(5):1–21.
[17] Riemer M. The Contextualized Feedback Intervention Theory: a theory of guided behavior
    change [master's thesis]. Nashville (TN): Vanderbilt University; 2003.
[18] Bickman L, Riemer M. Improving client outcomes through feedback to therapists: the theory.
    Presented at the 16th Annual Research Conference, A System of Care for Children's Mental
    Health: Expanding the Research Base. Tampa, FL; 2003.
[19] Carver CS, Scheier MF. Attention and self-regulation: a control therapy approach to human
    behavior. New York: Springer Press; 1981.
[20] Klein HJ. An integrated control theory model of work motivation. Acad Manage Rev 1989;
    14(3):150–72.
[21] Miller GA, Galanter E, Pribram KH. Plans and the structure of behavior. New York: Henry Holt
    and Co.; 1960.
[22] Powers WT. Behavior: the control of perception. Chicago: Aldine Publishing Co.; 1973.
[23] Taylor MS, Fisher CD, Ilgen DR. Individuals' reactions to performance feedback in or-
    ganizations: a control theory perspective. Res Personnel Human Resour Manage 1984;2:
    81–124.
[24] Hollenbeck JR, Williams CR, Klein HJ. An empirical examination of the antecedents of com-
    mitment to difficult goals. J Appl Psychol 1989;74(1):18–23.

[25] Hollenbeck JR, Klein HJ. Goal commitment and the goal-setting process: problems, prospects, and proposals for future research. J Appl Psychol 1987;72(2):212–20.

[26] Heneman HG, Schwab DP. Evaluation of research on expectancy theory predictions of employee performance. Psychol Bull 1972;78(1):1–9.

[27] Bandura A. Self-efficacy mechanism in human agency. Am Psychol 1982;37(2):122–47.

[28] Bandura A. Self-efficacy: the exercise of control. New York: W.H. Freeman & Co.; 1997.

[29] Ford M, editor. Motivating humans. Newbury Park (CA): Sage Publications; 1992.

[30] Jaen CR, Stange KC, Nutting PA. Competing demands of primary care: a model for the delivery of clinical preventative services. J Fam Pract 1994;38:166–71.

[31] Klinkman MS. Competing demands in psychosocial care: a model for the identification and treatment of depressive disorders in primary care. Gen Hosp Psychiat 1997;19(2):98–111.

[32] Henggeler SW, Schoenwald SK, Liao JG, Letourneau EJ, Edwards DL. Transporting efficacious treatments to field settings: the link between supervisory practices and therapist fidelity in MST programs. J Clin Child Psychol 2002;31(2):155–67.

[33] Addis ME. Methods for disseminating research products and increasing evidence-based practice: promises, obstacles, and future directions. Clin Psychol-Sci Pr 2002;9:367–78.

[34] Simpson DD. A conceptual framework for transferring research to practice. J Subst Abuse Treat 2002;22(4):171–82.

[35] Kluger AN, DeNisi A. The effects of feedback interventions on performance: a historical review, a meta-analysis, and a preliminary feedback intervention theory. Psychol Bull 1996;119(2):254–84.

[36] Lambert MJ, Hansen NB, Finch AE. Patient-focused research: using patient outcome data to enhance treatment effects. J Consult Clin Psych 2001;69(2):159–72.

[37] Howard KI, Moras K, Brill PL, Martinovich Z, Lutz W. Evaluation of psychotherapy: efficacy, effectiveness, and patient progress. Am Psychol 1996;51(10):1059–64.

[38] Lutz W. Patient-focused psychotherapy research and individual treatment progress as scientific groundwork for an empirically based clinical practice. Psychother Res 2002;12(3):251–72.

[39] Ilgen DR, Fisher CD, Taylor SM. Consequences of individual feedback on behavior in organizations. J Appl Psychol 1979;64(4):349–71.

[40] Hibbard JH. Use of outcome data by purchasers and consumers: new strategies and new dilemmas. Int J Qual Health C 1998;10(6):503–8.

[41] London M. Job feedback: giving, seeking, and using feedback for performance improvement. Mahway (NJ): Lawrence Erlbaum; 1997.

[42] Wilson C, Boni N, Hogg A. The effectiveness of task classification, positive reinforcement and corrective feedback in changing courtesy among police staff. J Organ Behav Manage 1997;17(1):65–99.

[43] Blanton H, Pelham BW, DeHart T, Carvallo M. Overconfidence as dissonance reduction. J Exp Soc Psychol 2001;37(5):373–85.

[44] Sherman DK, Cohen GL. Accepting threatening information: self-affirmation and the reduction of defensive biases. Curr Dir Psychol Sci 2002;11(4):119–22.

[45] Festinger L. A theory of cognitive dissonance. Evanston (IL): Row Peterson; 1957.

[46] Wicklund RA, Brehm JW. Perspectives on cognitive dissonance. Hillsdale (NJ): Lawrence Erlbaum Associates; 1976.

[47] Aronson E. Dissonance, hypocrisy, and the self-concept. In: Harmon-Jones E, Mills J, editors. Cognitive dissonance: progress on a pivotal theory in social psychology. Washington, DC: American Psychological Association; 1999. p. 103–26.

[48] Harmon-Jones E, Mills J. Cognitive dissonance- progress on a pivotal theory in social psychology. Washington, DC: American Psychological Association; 1999.

[49] Locke EA, Latham GP. Building a practically useful theory of goal setting and task motivation. Am Psychol 2002;57(9):705–17.

[50] Weiner B. An attributional theory of achievement motivation and emotion. Psychol Rev 1985;92(4):548–73.

[51] Prochaska JO. Strong and weak principles for progressing from precontemplation to action on the basis of twelve problem behaviors. Health Psychol 1994;13(1):47–51.

[52] Prochaska JO, Velicer WF, Rossi JS, Goldstein MG, Marcus BH, Rakowski W, et al. Stages of change and decisional balance for 12 problem behaviors. Health Psychol 1994;13(1):39–46.

[53] Levesque DA, Prochaska JM, Prochaska JO, Dewart SR, Hamby L, Weeks WB. Organizational stages and processes of change for continuous quality improvement in health care. Consult Psychol J Prac Res 2001;53(3):139–53.

[54] Velicer WF, DiClemente CC, Prochaska JO, Brandenburg N. Decisional balance measure for assessing and predicting smoking status. J Pers Soc Psychol 1985;48(5):1279–89.

[55] Bandura A. Health promotion from the perspective of social cognitive theory. Psychol Health 1998;13:623–49.

[56] Green LW, Kreuter MW. Health promotion planning: an educational and environmental approach. Mountain View (CA): Mayfield Publishing Co.; 1991.

[57] Oxman AD, Thomson MA, Davis D, Haynes BR. No magic bullets: a systematic review of 102 trials of intervention to improve professional practice. Can Med Assoc J 1995;153(10): 1423–31.

ELSEVIER
SAUNDERS

Child Adolesc Psychiatric Clin N Am
14 (2005) 255–271

CHILD AND
ADOLESCENT
PSYCHIATRIC CLINICS
OF NORTH AMERICA

Measuring Provider Attitudes Toward Evidence-Based Practice: Consideration of Organizational Context and Individual Differences

Gregory A. Aarons, PhD[a,b,*]

[a]Child and Adolescent Services Research Center, 3020 Children's Way, MC-5033, San Diego, CA 92123-4282, USA
[b]Departments of Psychiatry and Psychology, McGill Hall, 9500 Gilman Drive, University of California San Diego, School of Medicine, La Jolla, CA 92093, USA

There is increasing concern that technologies for treating child and adolescent mental health disorders be evidence based [1–7]. Evidence-based practices (EBPs) for youths and families are a subset of child and adolescent interventions with empirical support for their efficacy or effectiveness, and recent definitions include not only scientific rigor but also clinical judgment and consumer preference [8]. Although large-scale studies have found that system changes may fail to improve service outcomes [9], interventions with demonstrated efficacy or effectiveness hold promise in regard to improving outcomes for youths and families who receive mental health services [10–12].

The building momentum in the United States for the dissemination and adoption of EBP in private and public mental health service settings is bringing pressure on providers to adopt EBP, ready or not. The sources of such pressure for mental health service providers include government agencies, mental health authorities, agency directors, health management organizations, insurance companies, supervisors, peers, and consumers [13]. Little is known about attitudes that may facilitate or impede adoption of EBP among behavioral health service providers, however.

This work was supported by National Institute of Mental Health grant number MH01695. The Evidence-Based Practice Attitude Scale is available from the author.
* Child and Adolescent Services Research Center, 3020 Children's Way, MC-5033, San Diego, CA 92123-4282.
E-mail address: gaarons@ucsd.edu or gaarons@casrc.org

Invoking attitude change as a way to change behavior has shown promise. For example, in medical settings, experiential learning, including clinical experience, is more effective in changing attitudes compared with didactic learning [14,15]. This parallels marketing studies that demonstrate greater attitude change and attitude-behavior consistency for product experience versus advertising alone [16]. The sequencing and affective quality of information provided to change attitudes also must be considered. For example, when a large amount of information is to be provided, information that is affectively congruent is best presented early in the sequence [17]. There is a need to refine measurement to better understand the relationship of beliefs, attitudes, and behavior [18], and little attention has been given to measurement of mental heath provider attitudes toward adoption of EBP.

In contrast to mechanical innovations and technologic innovations such as computer hardware or software, behavioral health service technologies are considered to be "soft" technologies. Soft technologies are especially vulnerable to characteristics of the individual adopter and the implementation context for faithful implementation [10,19]. Individual providers bring their own characteristics, including such factors as education, training, beliefs, and personality. The context of mental health services also varies and includes the structures, processes, and procedures of organizations that can affect worker attitudes. Provider characteristics and organizational context are important in understanding how to move EBPs effectively into real world settings, and attitudes likely play a role.

Attitudes toward organizational change have been shown to be important in the dynamics of innovation [20]. Organizational readiness to change encompasses structures (eg, availability of computer resources) and processes (eg, cohesion, pressure for change) that may be related to attitudes toward adoption of EBPs [21]. One qualitative study in the public sector that included stakeholders across organizational levels—from agency directors to consumers—found multiple factors that impact the acceptability and likelihood of implementation of EBPs in community mental health settings (eg, perceived fit of the EBP with current practice, organization, and staff priorities) [22]. Such factors are likely to be associated with attitudes toward adoption of EBPs. The study of attitudes is also important because individual provider attitudes toward adoption of EBPs vary with individual difference factors and organizational characteristics [23].

The role of attitudes in models of innovation acceptance

Attitudes toward innovation can be a facilitating or limiting factor in the dissemination and implementation of new technologies [24,25]. Attitudes can be a precursor to the decision of whether to try a new practice, and the affective component of attitudes can impact decision processes regarding innovation [25–27]. The conceptual model in Fig. 1 illustrates proposed roles for attitudes in EBP acceptance and provides a useful heuristic in two ways. First, it identifies

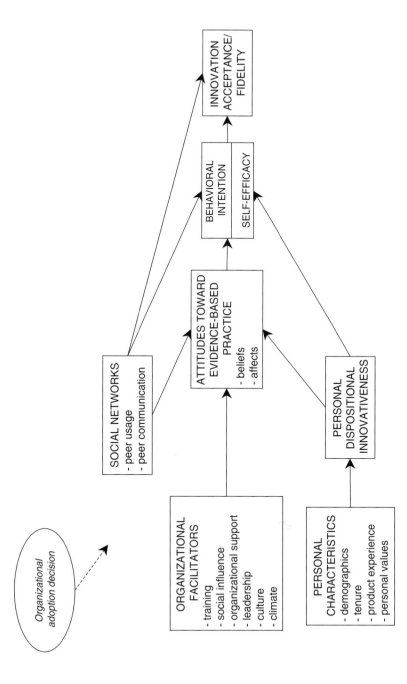

Fig. 1. Conceptual framework of the role of attitudes in innovation acceptance and evidence-based practice implementation in organizations. (*Adapted from* Frambach RT, Schillewaert N. Organizational innovation adoption: a multi-level framework of determinants and opportunities for future research. Journal of Business Research 2002;55:163–76; with permission.)

factors likely to influence attitudes toward EBP. Second, it illustrates the role of attitudes in acceptance of EBP. These factors can increase or decrease the likelihood that new technologies or services will be implemented as intended [25]. As shown in Fig. 1, attitudes toward adoption of EBP are proposed to be influenced by organizational facilitators, individual provider characteristics, provider dispositional innovativeness, and social networks. Attitudes are then proposed to be associated with behavioral intentions and self-efficacy and to affect innovation acceptance and fidelity with which EBPs are applied in practice. The constructs in this heuristic model are briefly described herein.

Organizational facilitators include training, social influences, organizational support for EBP, leadership, and organizational culture and climate that can increase or decrease the likelihood that new technologies or services will be implemented as intended [25]. Organizational support for innovation has not been well studied in human service agencies but can be defined as the extent to which employees perceive that they are supported in new ideas or in applying innovation [28]. Organizational support is believed to include support for creativity, tolerance of differences, and personal commitment [29].

Leadership affects many aspects of an organization's environment, including overall organizational functioning and team and individual functioning [30]. Leadership is important in effective operation of human service organizations, and good leadership is associated with higher levels of service provider organizational commitment and job satisfaction [31,32]. Leadership also influences provider ratings of working alliance in youth mental health programs through its influence on organizational climate [33].

Organizational culture can be defined as the implicit norms, values, shared behavioral expectations, and assumptions that guide behaviors of members of a work unit [34]. Organizational culture can impact how readily new technologies are considered and adopted in practice [35], and concern exists that public sector service organizations have cultures that resist innovation [36,37]. Technology transfer may be facilitated by adjusting an implementation plan to the culture of a human service agency, however [38]. For example, where programs have a conceptual adherence to certain principles of working with clients, new technologies or procedures might be framed as ancillary, rather than a replacement to current technologies being used. In human services, organizational culture influences provider attitudes, perceptions, and behaviors [39]. Carmazzi and Aarons [40] found that negative organizational culture was associated with providers' negative attitudes toward adoption of EBP, whereas positive culture was associated with openness to adoption of EBP.

Organizational climate refers to employees' perceptions and affective responses to their work environment [41–43]. Climate includes perceptions of job characteristics (eg, autonomy, variety, feedback, role clarity) and the work group (eg, cooperation, warmth, intimacy) [31]. Glisson and Hemmelgarn [44] demonstrated that organizational climate significantly impacted clinical outcomes for youth in publicly funded human services. Aarons et al [33] found that the effect of leadership on working alliance was mediated by organizational climate, and climate for innovation is a factor in human service organizational openness to change [45]. West [46] proposed four factors related to climate for innovation: vision, participative safety, task orientation, and support for innovation [47].

Social influence includes "processes by which individuals are affected by others' social construction of...events, ideas, objects, and behaviors and are subject to pressure to conform their behavior, attitudes, and beliefs to that social reality" [48]. Four social norms in the workplace are positively associated with group innovation: (1) support for creativity and risk taking, (2) teamwork, (3) speed of action, and (4) tolerance of mistakes [49]. Norms within workgroups can be influential in shaping behaviors, which can occur through social processes in organizations. Such social influence norms identify socially acceptable behavior in which adherence to rules provides social approval and rejection avoidance [50]. It follows that agencies with social processes that support innovation would be more likely to have employees likely to accept variation in work routines tied to EBP.

Personal characteristics include demographic factors, such as age, ethnicity, level of education, training, primary discipline, and amount of professional experience. These factors have been identified as potentially important in adoption of innovation. For example, factors such as level of education and level of professional experience have been found to be associated with attitudes toward adoption of EBP [23].

Personal dispositional innovativeness represents an individual's willingness and desire to experiment with new procedures, new tasks, or new ways of helping clients. Although organizational context and demand characteristics can impact staff innovativeness [46], individuals bring with them personality characteristics and behavior patterns. Personal dispositional characteristics of adaptability and willingness to lead change are associated with more positive attitudes toward adoption of EBP [51].

Social networks have to do with peer use of EBPs and communication about the EBPs, including the increase in perceived value and probability of adoption of an innovation as a critical mass of similar or interrelated organizations adopt the innovation [25,52]. It follows that as the number of mental health providers and agencies implementing an EBP increases and they have a positive experience, attitudes toward the EBP will become more favorable and the probability of additional providers and agencies adopting the EBP should increase.

Attitudes, along with behavioral intention and self-efficacy, often precede behavior and can predict behavior change [53–56]. In the heuristic model shown in Fig. 1, the effect of attitudes on innovation acceptance and fidelity is associated with behavioral intention and self-efficacy. It is likely, however, that additional factors (eg, provider conscientiousness) also come into play in determining overall provider effectiveness [57,58].

The way in which innovation acceptance is operationalized varies with the type of innovation. For EBPs, results of effectiveness trials suggest that successful translation of laboratory models into the field depends on maintaining fidelity to the intervention model. The extent to which an EBP is successful in generating expected outcomes likely is affected by the degree to which it is implemented correctly and by contextual influences [59,60].

As mentioned previously and in Fig. 1, attitudes are proposed to function in a complex context. For example, studies have shown that organizational culture and climate affect provider work attitudes, service quality, and outcomes [33,39,44]. Organizational context also can impact staff attitudes toward innovation [46]. Attitudes are part of a complex interaction of context, beliefs, intentions, and behavior [55]; however, little research to date has identified provider attitudes toward adoption of EBP. The next section describes proposed domains of attitudes toward adoption of EBP.

Four proposed domains of attitudes toward adoption of evidence-based practice

Four domains of attitudes to adoption of EBP have recently been identified, including attitudes related to the appeal of an EBP, requirements to adopt an EBP, openness to innovation in general, and perceived divergence between current work processes and those of the EBP.

Appeal of evidence-based practice

Studies of persuasion processes and provider self-efficacy support the notion that attitudes and attitude change are sensitive to the information source and the valence or appeal of information [50,61,62]. For example, providers are more at ease with information derived from colleagues in contrast to research articles or books [63,64]. This factor is important in considering the likely attractiveness of innovations including EBPs [25].

Requirements to adopt evidence-based practice

Attitudes toward requirements to change practice also vary from person to person. For example, a recent study found variability in provider attitudes and compliance with new required assessment practices for using a particular set of standardized measures [65]. Although some providers may be more or less compliant with required changes, individual and organizational variability can affect the degree to which innovations are adopted and sustained in practice [19,27].

Openness to innovation

Openness to change in general has been identified as an important component of workplace climate that can impact innovation in mental health service programs [45]. Openness to innovation is considered an important characteristic of staff in "learning organizations," and such organizations are more responsive and adaptive to contingencies [45,66–68]. Personal dispositional innovativeness represents one's general openness to innovation and willingness to experiment with new technologies [25]. This general openness is akin to the personality characteristic of openness [69]. Provider adaptability is also associated with more positive attitudes toward adoption of EBP [51]. General openness to innovation is not conditional on the appeal of an EBP, however.

Perceived divergence

Problems in dissemination and implementation of EBP are likely to occur when there is a perceived difference between current and new practices and current practice has a more positive valence. For example, mandated use of evidence-based assessment protocols is often perceived as incongruent or unneeded in clinical practice [65]. Interventions developed in academic or research-based settings may be perceived to lack real world clinical validity and utility. Even where systems are in place to make the use of an EBP relatively seamless, there may be perceived divergence.

To understand better the role of provider attitudes in adoption of EBP, reliable and valid measures of provider attitudes toward adoption of EBP are needed. The next section describes such a measure and summarizes preliminary findings.

The Evidence-based Practice Attitude Scale

The Evidence-based Practice Attitude Scale (EBPAS) is a brief (15-item) measure that assesses four general attitudes toward adoption of EBP (Table 1) [23]. The development of the scale was based on literature reviews, discussions with providers and researchers, item generation, data collection, and exploratory and confirmatory factor analyses. Reliability and validity analyses also were conducted and are summarized later [23].

The EBPAS consists of four theoretically derived subscales of attitudes toward adoption of EBP, including appeal, requirements, openness, divergence, and the EBPAS total scale score. The appeal scale represents the extent to which the provider would adopt an EBP if it were intuitively appealing, could be used correctly, or was being used by colleagues who were happy with it. The requirements scale assesses the extent to which the provider would adopt an EBP if it were required by an agency, supervisor, or state. The openness scale assesses the extent to which the provider is generally open to trying new interventions and would be willing to try or use EBPs. The divergence scale assesses the extent to which the provider perceives EBPs as not clinically useful and less important than clinical experience. The EBPAS total scale score represents one's global attitude toward adoption of EBP. The overall Cronbach's alpha reliability for the EBPAS is good (alpha = 0.77), and subscale alphas range from 0.90 to 0.59 [23].

Table 1
Evidence–based pratice attitude scale (EBPAS): items, factor loadings, Chronbach's alphas, and scoring

Item #	Scale	Factor loading	Alpha
	Scale 1: requirements		0.90
12	Agency required	0.99	
11	Supervisor required	0.88	
13	State required	0.78	
	Scale 2: appeal		0.80
10	Makes sense	0.89	
9	Intuitively appealing	0.83	
14	Colleages happy with therapy	0.56	
15	Enough training	0.55	
	Scale 3: openness		0.78
2	Will follow a treatment manual	0.61	
4	Will try therapy/interventions developed by researchers	0.81	
1	Like to use new therapy/interventions	0.62	
8	Would try therapy/interventions different than usual	0.66	
	Scale 4: divergence		0.59
5	Research-based treatments/interventions not useful	0.65	
7	Would not use manualized therapy/interventions	0.76	
6	Clinical experience more important	0.42	
3	Know better than researchers how to care for clients	0.34	
	EBPAS Total		0.77

Scoring the scales. The score for each subscale is created by computing a mean score for each set of items that load on a given subscale. For example, items 14, 15, and 16 constitute Scale 1. If there are missing data in your data set, computing means may be done allowing for one fewer item than makes up the scale.

Computing the total score. Only for the total score (not the individual scale scores), items from subscale 4 (divergence) must be reverse scored and the subscale score recomputed. After the reverse scoring is complete, a mean of the scale scores may be computed to yield the mean score for the total EBPAS.

You may contact Dr. Aarons by e-mail at: gaarons@casrc.org.

From Aarons GA. Mental health provider attitudes toward adoption of evidence–based practice: the evidence–based practice attitude scale. Mental Health Services Research 2004;6(2): 61–74; with permission.

Preliminary EBPAS validity analyses suggest that scale scores vary with important provider and organizational characteristics. For example, interns were more likely to score higher on appeal, openness, and total EBPAS scales, which indicated more openness to innovation compared with more experienced professionals. Interns also tended to score lower on the divergence scale, which indicated less perceived difference between EBP and usual practice compared with more experienced professionals [23].

Higher educational attainment was associated with higher scores on the EBPAS appeal dimension. Level of education and intern status overlap and are clearly related, but they represent qualitatively different aspects of a mental health care provider's professional developmental trajectory. This relationship suggests that although more professional education is associated with openness to EBPs, professional internships may be an especially opportune stage of a service provider's professional development in which to introduce and reinforce the value of the use of EBPs [23].This is congruent with studies that show that during pre-professional status, workers may be particularly predisposed to the acquisition of new practices [70–72].

In addition to provider characteristics, organizational characteristics were related to attitudes toward adoption of EBP. For example, providers who work in differing types of agencies endorsed different levels of attitudes to EBP. In contrast to outpatient clinic providers, providers who work in wraparound programs endorsed more open attitudes to adoption of EBP, and providers who work in case management programs were less open to adoption of EBPs. This result suggests that it is important to consider the programmatic context into which EBPs are to be disseminated and implemented [23].

Organizational structure and formalization of clinic procedures also should be considered regarding their effect on attitudes [19,73]. For example, providers who work in mental health programs with low levels of bureaucracy endorsed more positive attitudes to adoption of EBPs. Some programs institute policies regarding interventions to be used for specific problems or disorders. The presence of such policies acquaints providers with a higher degree of procedural specification that is similar to that required by many EBPs. Providers who work in programs with formalized practice policies endorsed more positive attitudes toward adoption of EBPs [23]. Although this finding may seem discordant with studies that reported that top-down models of imposing new procedures may engender resistance [65], the internal written policies noted were part of a culture of objectivism in considering how best to match interventions to presenting problems. Given these findings, it is important to determine if the relationship of provider attitudes, provider characteristics, and organizational characteristics can be understood better to facilitate EBP adoption.

Adopter characteristics and attitudes toward evidence-based practice

Regarding adoption of innovation, five groups have been delineated, including innovators, early adopters, the early majority, the late majority, and "laggards" [27]. Innovators are those who have curiosity and keen interest in new technologies. Early adopters are more cautious than innovators but are still willing to experiment when a new technology shows promise. The early majority is still more cautious, and they wait until some promise of a technology is shown through the experiences of early adopters. The late majority is even more cautious and risk averse, and they wait until there is ample evidence that the risks of adopting the technology are low and benefits are evident. Laggards, on the other hand, are unlikely to adopt a new technology unless it is absolutely necessary or an extremely convincing case has been made for adoption. For research on dissemination and implementation of particular EBPs, it is important to understand where a behavioral health care service provider resides along the adoption likelihood dimension and how to bridge the gap between adopter groups to promote diffusion and adoption of EBP [74].

Measurement of attitudes toward adoption of EBP may provide an index of likelihood of actual adoption and help to generate testable hypotheses. For example, providers who score high on the EBPAS appeal and openness scales might fall into the innovator or early adopter categories. In contrast, providers who score low on the EBPAS appeal, openness, and requirements scales and high on the divergence scale likely would fall into the late majority or laggard groups. As with the study of dissemination and implementation of EBP [75], however, the measurement of attitudes toward adoption of EBP and application to other models is in its infancy, and these hypotheses remain to be tested.

Learning organizations and incentives for change

EBP dissemination and implementation efforts should address attitudes of staff and specific operational contexts. Some providers and organizations may be poised to respond to environmental contingencies, such as changes in contracting and practice demands, whereas others may be less flexible regarding changes in policies or procedures. The notion of the organization as an adaptive system extends the research on learning organizations and holds promise as an explanatory model of change in behavioral health services [76]. The development of a learning organization depends not only on adaptive processes but also on cultivating positive provider attitudes and having technology and structure that promote communication and change.

Future directions

EBPs hold the promise of improving a provider's ability to help clients and patients and improve cost effectiveness [10]. To reach providers, marketing strategies that present new interventions as appealing, effective, and in demand with colleagues and from consumers may be helpful in promoting positive attitudes toward adopting EBPs. Another likely lever for increasing positive provider attitudes toward adoption of EBPs is the notion that special expertise derived from learning an EBP can improve self-perceptions of professional accomplishment and self-efficacy to effectively work with clients, gain employment, and promote one's practice.

Several areas are ripe for research on the contribution of attitudes to dissemination and implementation (DI) of EBPs. It is important to identify additional factors associated with improving attitudes toward adoption of EBPs, including identifying those who are most likely to seek out and use EBPs and addressing concerns of those who are not. Researchers often perceive EBPs as necessary for effective service delivery, but providers may be more reserved and cautious about what it means to adopt a new practice [65]. While frequently juggling overwhelming clinical and administrative responsibilities, taking on new and different job tasks may be seen as a difficult endeavor with questionable rewards. The impact of mental health clinic culture and climate on attitudes toward EBP should be considered [39]. For example, an organizational culture that engenders negative attitudes to change suggests the need to address resistance not only to EBP but also to organizational change in general. Including staff in discussions about changes in practice and how EBP is congruent with current approaches may decrease perceived divergence between current and new practice and facilitate change [68].

Little is known regarding the interaction of organizational characteristics and provider characteristics when an EBP is implemented. For example, organizational culture provides norms for behavior within an organization. If attitudes toward adoption of EBP are weak and culture is strong, then the effect of culture may overpower attitudes. Strong attitudes can be congruent or incongruent with organizational norms, however [77]. To the degree that attitudes toward adoption of EBP are at odds with organizational norms and proposed organizational change, staff may perceive the climate as stressful, and poor work attitudes, poor job performance, and staff turnover may result [78,79]. This is just one example of how organizational and individual factors can interact, and more study of such factors is needed.

The effectiveness of implementation efforts likely will be impacted by provider attitudes toward EBP, the specific type of EBP, organizational climate for innovation, and the fit between personal values and those of the organization. This "innovation-values fit" can be maximized by providing a strong implementation climate, ensuring skill in the innovation, providing incentives for its use, and removing obstacles to use of the innovation [80]. An organization can provide incentives for employees through praise, encouragement by supervisors, and the provision of tangible and valued rewards [28]. Obstacles can be removed by including participative decision making about the innovation, allowing ample time for learning about the innovation, and responding to questions and complaints about the innovation by employees [28,80]. A good innovation-values fit also can be facilitated through strong commitment to and support of the innovation by the organization, communication and information sharing throughout the organization, the inclusion of "champions" or respected individuals who actively promote the innovation, and the existence of a strong social network that allows for increased positive interaction among employees [25,28,81].

To promote diffusion of EBP, strategies from marketing and organizational literatures could be considered. Innovators and early adopters are more likely to have positive attitudes toward innovation and be less concerned with how current behaviors diverge from those required for the new technology [74]. Innovators and early adopters of EBPs could be encouraged to communicate with other more reticent mental health care professionals. More attention should be given to bridging the gap between adopter groups [27,74]. In particular, the communication and spread of enthusiasm and positive experiences of innovators and early adopters could be facilitated. The most effective means by which such communication takes place should be identified and exploited. Identification of factors that promote or inhibit adoption of EBP improves our ability to tailor implementation efforts to the characteristics and needs of specific mental health service providers and organizations.

The degree to which provider attitudes toward adoption of EBP are important in models of DI remains to be tested. The long history of attitudes as a factor in behavior change suggests that they will contribute to understanding and improving the EBP DI process. Currently, models of DI should include attitudes as one factor that may influence EBP acceptance, fidelity, and outcomes.

Acknowledgments

The author thanks the program managers, clinicians, and case managers who participated in the scale development study.

Appendix. Evidence-based practice attitude scale

The following questions ask about your feelings about using new types of therapy, interventions, or treatments. Manualized therapy refers to any intervention that has specific guidelines and/or components that are outlined in a manual and/or are to be followed in a structured or predetermined way.

Fill in the circle indicating the extent to which you agree with each item using the following scale:

Evidence-based practice attitude scale

The following questions ask about your feelings about using new types of therapy, interventions, or treatments. Manualized therapy refers to any intervention that has specific guidelines and/or components that are outlined in a manual and/or that are to be followed in a structured/predetermined way.

Fill in the circle indicating the extent to which you agree with each item using the following scale:

0	1	2	3	4
Not at All	To a Slight Extent	To a Moderate Extent	To a Great Extent	To a Very Great Extent

	0	1	2	3	4
1. I like to use new types of therapy/interventions to help my clients............................	○	○	○	○	○
2. I am willing to try new types of therapy/interventions even if I have to follow a treatment manual..	○	○	○	○	○
3. I know better than academic researchers how to care for my clients............................	○	○	○	○	○
4. I am willing to use new and different types of therapy/interventions developed by researchers..	○	○	○	○	○
5. Research based treatments/interventions are not clinically useful...............................	○	○	○	○	○
6. Clinical experience is more important than using manualized therapy/treatment............	○	○	○	○	○
7. I would not use manualized therapy/interventions...	○	○	○	○	○
8. I would try a new therapy/intervention even if it were very different from what I am used to doing..	○	○	○	○	○

For questions 9-15: If you received training in a therapy or intervention that was new to you, how likely would you be to adopt it if:

	0	1	2	3	4
9. it was intuitively appealing?..	○	○	○	○	○
10. it "made sense" to you?..	○	○	○	○	○
11. it was required by your supervisor?...	○	○	○	○	○
12. it was required by your agency?...	○	○	○	○	○
13. it was required by your state?..	○	○	○	○	○
14. it was being used by colleagues who were happy with it?......................................	○	○	○	○	○
15. you felt you had enough training to use it correctly?...	○	○	○	○	○

References

[1] Hebert R. NIMH strategies for moving evidence-based mental illness treatments from laboratory to real-world therapies. Observer 2003;16:21–4.

[2] Hoagwood K, Olin S. The NIMH blueprint for change report: research priorities in child and adolescent mental health. J Am Acad Child Adolesc Psychiatry 2002;41:760–7.

[3] Jensen PS. The next generation is overdue [commentary]. J Am Acad Child Adolesc Psychiatry 2003;42:527–30.

[4] Kazdin AE, Weisz JR. Identifying and developing empirically supported child and adolescent treatments. J Consult Clin Psychol 1998;66:19–36.

[5] National Institute of Mental Health. Bridging science and service (No. 99–4353). Bethesda: National Institutes of Health; 1999.

[6] National Institute of Mental Health. What do we know about implementing evidence-based practices (EBPs) and where can we go from here? Bethesda: National Institutes of Health; 2002.

[7] National Institute of Mental Health. Translating behavioral science into action: report of the national advisory mental health council behavioral science workgroup (No. 00–4699). Bethesda: National Institutes of Health; 2000.

[8] Institute of Medicine, Institute of Medicine Committee on the Quality of Health Care in America. Crossing the quality chasm: a new health system for the 21st century. Washington DC: National Academy Press; 2001.

[9] Bickman L. The evaluation of a children's mental health managed care demonstration. J Ment Health Adm 1996;23:7–15.

[10] Barnoski R. Outcome evaluation of Washington State's research-based programs for juvenile offenders. Olympia (WA): Washington State Institute for Public Policy; 2004.

[11] Burns BJ. Children and evidence-based practice. Psychiatr Clin North Am 2003;26:955–70.

[12] Hoagwood K, Burns BJ, Kiser L, Ringeisen H, Schoenwald SK. Evidence-based practice in child and adolescent mental health services. Psychiatr Serv 2001;52:1179–89.

[13] Essock SM, Goldman HH, Van Tosh L, et al. Evidence-based practices: setting the context and responding to concerns. Psychiatr Clin North Am 2003;26:919–38.

[14] Peters AS, Schimpfhauser FT, Cheng J, Daly SL, et al. Effect of a course in cancer prevention on students' attitudes and clinical behavior. J Med Educ 1987;62:592–600.

[15] Warburg MM, Cleary PD, Rohman ME, Barnes HN, et al. Residents' attitudes, knowledge, and behavior regarding diagnosis and treatment of alcoholism. J Med Educ 1987;62:497–503.

[16] Smith RE, Swinyard WR. Attitude-behavior consistency: the impact of product trial versus advertising. J Mark Res 1983;20:257–67.

[17] Jacoby J, Morrin M, Jaccard J, Gurhan Z, Kuss A, Maheswaran D. Mapping attitude formation as a function of information input: online processing models of attitude formation. Journal of Consumer Psychology 2002;12:21–34.

[18] Jaccard J, Radecki C, Wilson T, Dittus P. Methods for identifying consequential beliefs: implications for understanding attitude strength. In: Petty RE, Krosnick JA, editors. Attitude strength: antecedents and consequences. Ohio State University series on attitudes and persuasion. Hillsdale (NJ): Lawrence Erlbaum Associates Inc.; 1995. p. 337–59.

[19] Glisson C. The organizational context of children's mental health services. Clin Child Fam Psychol Rev 2002;5:233–53.

[20] Dunham RB, Grube JA, Gardner DG, Pierce JL. The development of an attitude toward change instrument. Presented at the 49th Annual Meeting of the Academy of Management. Washington, DC, August 14–16, 1989.

[21] Lehman WEK, Greener JM, Simpson DD. Assessing organizational readiness for change. J Subst Abuse Treat 2002;22:197–209.

[22] Hurlburt M, Knapp P. The new consumers of evidence-based practices: reflections of providers and families. Data matters, special issue number 6. Washington, DC: National Technical Assistance Center for Children's Mental Health: Georgetown University Center for Child and Human Development; 2003. p. 21–3.

[23] Aarons GA. Mental health provider attitudes toward adoption of evidence-based practice: the evidence-based practice attitude scale. Ment Health Serv Res 2004;6:61–72.

[24] Damanpour F. Organizational innovation: a meta-analysis of effects of determinants and moderators. Acad Manage J 1991;34:555–90.

[25] Frambach RT, Schillewaert N. Organizational innovation adoption: a multi-level framework of determinants and opportunities for future research. Journal of Business Research 2002;55: 163–76.

[26] Candel MJJM, Pennings JME. Attitude-based models for binary choices: a test for choices involving an innovation. J Econ Psychol 1999;20:547–69.

[27] Rogers EM. Diffusion of innovations. 4th edition. New York: The Free Press; 1995.

[28] Ash J. Organizational factors that influence information technology diffusion in academic health sciences centers. J Am Med Inform Assoc 1997;4:102–11.

[29] Siegel SM, Kaemmerer WF. Measuring the perceived support for innovation in organizations. J Appl Psychol 1978;63:553–62.

[30] Bass BM, Avolio BJ, Jung DI, Berson Y. Predicting unit performance by assessing transformational and transactional leadership. J Appl Psychol 2003;88:207–18.

[31] Glisson C. The effect of leadership on workers in human service organizations. Adm Soc Work 1989;13:99–116.

[32] Glisson C, Durick M. Predictors of job satisfaction and organizational commitment in human service organizations. Adm Sci Q 1988;33:61–81.

[33] Aarons GA, Woodbridge M, Carmazzi A. Examining leadership, organizational climate and service quality in a children's system of care. In: Proceedings of the 15th Annual Research Conference. A system of care for children's mental health: examining the research base. Tampa: University of South Florida, Louis de la Parte Florida Mental Health Institute, Research and Training Center for Children's Mental Health; 2003. p. 15–8.

[34] Cooke RA, Rousseau DM. Behavioral norms and expectations: a quantitative approach to the assessment of organizational culture. Group and Organization Studies 1988;13:245–73.

[35] Hemmelgarn AL, Glisson C, Dukes D. Emergency room culture and the emotional support component of family-centered care. Child Health Care 2001;30:93–110.

[36] Backer TE, David SL, Soucy GE, editors. Reviewing the behavioral science knowledge base on technology transfer. (NIDA research monograph 155, NIH Publication No. 95–4035.). Rockville: National Institute on Drug Abuse; 1995.

[37] Diamond MA. Innovation and diffusion of technology: a human process. Consulting Psychology Journal: Practice and Research 1996;48:221–9.

[38] Keller DS, Galanter M. Technology transfer of network therapy to community-based addictions counselors. J Subst Abuse Treat 1999;16:183–9.

[39] Glisson C, James LR. The cross-level effects of culture and climate in human service teams. Journal of Organizational Behavior 2002;23:767–94.

[40] Carmazzi A, Aarons GA. Organizational culture and attitudes toward adoption of evidence-based practice. Presented at the NAMSHPD Research Institute's 2003 Conference on State Mental Health Agency Services Research, Program Evaluation, and Policy. Baltimore, February 10, 2003.

[41] Joyce WF, Slocum JW. Climate discrepancy: refining the concepts of psychological and organizational climate. Hum Relat 1982;35:951–71.

[42] Sells SB, James LR. Organizational climate. In: Nesselroade JR, Cattell RB, editors. Handbook of multivariate experimental psychology: perspectives on individual differences. 2nd edition. New York: Plenum Press; 1988. p. 915–37.

[43] Srivastava SK, Bathla A. Correlational study of organizational climate and work adjustment among industrial workers. Social Science International 1996;12:52–60.

[44] Glisson C, Hemmelgarn A. The effects of organizational climate and interorganizational coordination on the quality and outcomes of children's service systems. Child Abuse Negl 1998;22: 401–21.

[45] Anderson NR, West MA. Measuring climate for work group innovation: development and validation of the team climate inventory. Journal of Organizational Behavior 1998;19:235–58.

[46] West MA. The social psychology of innovation in groups. In: West MA, Farr JL, editors. Innovation and creativity at work: psychological and organizational strategies. Oxford (UK): John Wiley & Sons; 1990. p. 309–33.

[47] West MA, Anderson NR. Innovation in top management teams. J Appl Psychol 1996;81: 680–93.

[48] Lewis LK, Seibold DR. Innovation modification during intraorganizational adoption. Acad Manage Rev 1993;18:322–54.

[49] O'Reilly CA, Caldwell DF. The impact of normative social influence and cohesiveness on task perceptions and attitudes: a social information processing approach. Journal of Occupational Psychology 1985;58:193–206.

[50] Cialdini RB, Bator RJ, Guadagno RE. Normative influences in organizations. In: Thompson LL, Levine JM, Messick DM, editors. Shared cognition in organizations: the management of knowledge. Mahwah (NJ): Lawrence Erlbaum Associates; 1999. p. 195–211.

[51] Aarons GA. Service worker attitudes toward adoption of empirically supported treatments. Presented at the NASMHPD Research Institute's 2003 Conference on State Mental Health Agency Services Research, Program Evaluation, and Policy. Baltimore, February 10, 2003.

[52] Kraut RE, Rice RE, Cool C, Fish RS. Varieties of social influence: the role of utility and norms in the success of a new communication medium. Organization Science 1998;9:437–53.

[53] Bandura A. Self-efficacy mechanism in human agency. Am Psychol 1982;37:122–47.

[54] Bandura A. Growing primacy of human agency in adaptation and change in the electronic era. European Psychologist 2002;7:2–16.

[55] Fishbein M, Azjen I. Belief, attitude, intentions, and behavior: an introduction to theory and research. Reading (MA): Addison-Wesley; 1975.

[56] Fishbein M, Hennessy M, Yzer M, Douglas J. Can we explain why some people do and some people do not act on their intentions? Psychology Health and Medicine 2003;8:3–18.

[57] Mount MK, Barrick MR, Stewart GL. Five-factor model of personality and performance in jobs involving interpersonal interactions. Human Performance 1998;11:145–65.

[58] Witt L, Burke L, Barrick M, Mount M. The interactive effects of conscientiousness and agreeableness on job performance. J Appl Psychol 2002;87:164–9.

[59] Detrich R. Increasing treatment fidelity by matching interventions to contextual variables within the educational setting. School Psych Rev 1999;28:608–20.

[60] Schoenwald SK, Henggeler SW, Brondino MJ, Rowland MD. Multisystemic therapy: monitoring treatment fidelity. Fam Process 2000;39:83–103.

[61] Tormala ZL, Petty RE. What doesn't kill me makes me stronger: the effects of resisting persuasion on attitude certainty. J Pers Soc Psychol 2002;83:1298–313.

[62] Watkins M. Principles of persuasion. Negotiation Journal 2001;17:115–37.

[63] Cohen L, Sargent M, Sechrest L. Use of psychotherapy research by professional psychologists. Am Psychol 1986;41:198–206.

[64] Morrow-Bradley C, Elliott R. Utilization of psychotherapy research by practicing psychotherapists. Am Psychol 1986;41:188–97.

[65] Garland AF, Kruse M, Aarons GA. Clinicians and outcome measurement: what's the use? J Behav Health Serv Res 2003;30:393–405.

[66] Birleson P. Turning child and adolescent mental-health services into learning organizations. Clin Child Psychol Psychiatry 1999;4:265–74.

[67] Fiol CM, Lyles MA. Organizational learning. Acad Manage Rev 1985;10:803–13.

[68] Garvin DA. Building a learning organization. Harv Bus Rev 1993;71:78–91.

[69] McCrae RR, Costa PT. Validation of the five-factor model of personality across instruments and observers. J Pers Soc Psychol 1987;52:81–90.

[70] Day E, Arthur W, Gettman D. Knowledge structures and the acquisition of a complex skill. J Appl Psychol 2001;86:1022–33.

[71] Klimoski R, Mohammed S. Team mental model: construct or metaphor? J Manage 1994;20: 403–37.

[72] Rentsch JR, Klimoski RJ. Why do great minds think alike? Antecedents of team member schema agreement. Journal of Organizational Behavior 2001;22:107–20.

[73] Glisson C. Structure and technology in human service organizations. In: Hasenfeld Y, editor. Human services as complex organizations. Thousand Oaks (CA): Sage Publications; 1992. p. 184–202.

[74] Moore GA. Crossing the chasm: marketing and selling high-tech products to mainstream customers. New York: HarperCollins Publishers; 2002.

[75] Schoenwald SK, Sheidow AJ, Letourneau EJ, Liao JG. Transportability of multisystemic therapy: evidence for multilevel influences. Ment Health Serv Res 2003;5:223–39.

[76] Jankowicz D. From learning organization to adaptive organization. Management Learning 2000; 31:471–90.

[77] Harris SG, Mossholder KW. The affective implications of perceived congruence with culture dimensions during organizational transformation. Journal of Management 1996;22:527–47.

[78] Baron JN, Hannan MT, Burton MD. Labor pains: change in organizational models and employee turnover in young, high-tech firms. American Journal of Sociology 2001;106:960–1012.

[79] Gill S, Greenberg MT, Vazquez A. Changes in the service delivery model and home visitors' job satisfaction and turnover in an Early Head Start program. Infant Mental Health Journal 2002;23: 182–96.

[80] Klein KJ, Sorra JS. The challenge of innovation implementation. Acad Manage Rev 1996;21: 1055–80.

[81] Pullig C, Maxham JGI, Hair Jr JF. Salesforce automation systems: an exploratory examination of organizational factors associated with effective implementation and salesforce productivity. Journal of Business Research 2002;55:401–15.

ELSEVIER
SAUNDERS

Child Adolesc Psychiatric Clin N Am
14 (2005) 273–296

CHILD AND
ADOLESCENT
PSYCHIATRIC CLINICS
OF NORTH AMERICA

Using and Teaching Evidence-Based Medicine: The Duke University Child and Adolescent Psychiatry Model

John S. March, MD, MPH*, Allan Chrisman, MD,
Alfiee Breland-Noble, PhD, Kelly Clouse, MD,
Richard D'Alli, MD, Helen Egger, MD,
Pat Gammon, PhD, Marta Gazzola, MD, Anne Lin, MD,
Christian Mauro, PhD, Aasim Rana, MD,
Himabindu Ravi, MD, Madhanika Srirama, MD,
Hansen Su, MD, Grace Thrall, MD, Polly van de Velde, MSW
The Duke Pediatric Psychiatry EBM Seminar Team

*Department of Psychiatry and Behavioral Sciences, Duke Child and Family Study Center,
Duke University Medical Center, 718 Rutherford Street (DUMC 3527), Durham, NC 27710, USA*

Imagine that you are attending a seminar in evidence-based medicine (EBM) with about 20 other mental health professionals. About half of those in attendance are child and adolescent psychiatry trainees. The rest are faculty members split between child and adolescent psychiatry, medical psychology, and social work. The participants are engaged in an animated discussion about the treatment of children with tic disorders. The article being discussed, which was identified and retrieved using an Internet search at the start of the seminar, asks whether clonidine alone or in combination with a psychostimulant reduces attention-deficit/hyperactivity disorder (ADHD) symptoms or tics in children with a tic disorder and ADHD. The trainees, one of whom generated the question from a patient care experience, are considering whether the study design is valid, what the sample looks like, whether there is a significant effect of treatment, how big that effect is relative to clinical need, and whether there are modifying factors that would make the article more or less relevant to the care of the patient who

This study was supported by NIMH grants 1 K24 MHO1557 and 1 P30 MH066386-01A1 (to J.S. March).

* Corresponding author.
E-mail address: jsmarch@acpub.duke.edu (J.S. March).

prompted the question in the first place. In doing so, the trainees skimmed the abstract, carefully read the methods section, and went to a table in the results section to identify the response rates. Clinical issues, including doctor and patient preferences that might influence the choice of treatment, occupy a prominent place in the discussion. Faculty members chime in, but trainees lead the discussion. The whole process of "keeping up with the literature," including completing a critically appraised topic (CAT), was accomplished in less than 30 minutes.

As used here, EBM is defined as a set of processes that facilitate the conscientious, explicit, and judicious integration of individual clinical expertise with the best available external clinical evidence from systematic research in making decisions about the care of individual patients [1,2]. Most conventional approaches to understanding the scientific foundation of medical practice typically involve groups of experts asking whether there is or is not evidence [3–5]. In contrast, EBM focuses not only on grading the strength of the evidence but also on the processes and tools that are necessary for clinicians to continually upgrade their knowledge and skills for those problems encountered in daily practice. From the standpoint of training, EBM encourages trainees to develop skills and habits of critical thinking that are essential to life-long learning. Although EBM has become the standard heuristic for teaching and clinical practice in other areas of medicine, it is just now beginning to make inroads into psychiatry and has had little or no impact in academic psychology [2,6]. This article, authored by members of the Duke Pediatric Psychiatry EBM Seminar Team, (1) describes EBM as applied to the training of child and adolescent psychiatrists in the Division of Child and Adolescent Psychiatry, Department of Psychiatry at Duke University Medical Center; (2) presents a simplified discussion of EBM as a technology for training and patient care; (3) discusses the basic principles and procedures for teaching EBM in the setting of a multidisciplinary training program; and (4) briefly mentions two training and research initiatives that are furthered by incorporating EBM.

The Duke Pediatric Psychiatry Evidence-Based Medicine Seminar

First established over 10 years ago, the Pediatric Psychiatry EBM Seminar at Duke is consciously multidisciplinary, with participation from senior researchers, attending physicians, psychologists, social workers, child psychiatry fellows, and general psychiatry residents. The seminar is held each week on a Wednesday morning for 1.5 hours. At the beginning of each academic year, seminar participants review the EBM textbook by Sackett and colleagues [1] from beginning to end. The intent is to build the basic concepts and skills necessary for evidence-based practice. Selected materials from the *Journal of the American Medical Association* users' guides to EBM [7] and the EBM textbook by Gray [2] are provided to supplement the basic text. Advanced trainees typically lead the discussion at the beginning of each year, with faculty setting the agenda and ensuring that the focus stays on EBM. After basic skills are in place, the focus turns to polling and evaluating the literature based on clinical questions that arise directly from the patient care experiences of seminar participants.

In a seminal article entitled "Why I Don't Attend Case Conferences" that is still worth reading 30 years after its publication, the distinguished psychologist and psychiatric taxonomist Paul Meehl [8] wrote

> I remind the reader that a psychiatric case conference involves the welfare of patients and their families. ... I am deeply offended by the intellectual mediocrity of what transpires in most case conferences. ... The ignorance, errors, scientific fallacies, clinical carelessness, and slovenly mental habits...have—sometimes dramatically—an adverse impact upon human lives.

In most "journal club" exercises, an article is proposed by one of the faculty, read in advance, and one of the trainees takes on the unenviable job of summarizing the article (as though no one read it beforehand) while the rest sit around bored silly. The trainees then listen to the faculty discuss the article from the point of view of best-practice standards for patient care. In perusing the article, most of the participants will have read only the abstract, introduction, and discussion sections, skipping the methods and results and uninteresting and difficult to understand. Unless the discussion is explicitly focused on research methods—anathema to most trainees and clinical faculty—little consideration usually is given to whether the conclusions drawn by the investigators (or for that matter, the faculty) are valid for their intended purpose. Given that the focus is on opinion, not data, it is a rare, bold student who will offer a contradictory opinion. Many if not most of the articles chosen will be review articles or book chapters that lack even the most rudimentary attempts to systematically assess existing knowledge. Absent a focus on critical appraisal of the literature and subsequent integration of the evidence with clinical judgment, is it any wonder that tension almost always exists between the "evidence" and clinical experience, with some decrying the lack of relevance of the literature and others complaining that no one pays any attention to the evidence?

We presume that Paul Meehl, who preferred to attend case conferences in neurology to those in psychiatry or psychology, would be delighted to sit in on our EBM seminar, which although the diseases differ, is not materially different from EBM as applied in other areas of medicine [9]. Based in epidemiology, especially Bayesian approaches to estimating probability, we focus on using all available sources of information to give the best possible odds of a successful outcome, whether for diagnosis or treatment. In so doing, trainees (and faculty) master an easy-to-learn set of guidelines for accessing and evaluating an ever-involving and increasingly complex medical literature (eg, our EBM seminar recently spent 2 months applying the guidelines for establishing causality to pharmacogenetics in psychiatry). In turn, EBM provides a mechanism for "keeping up" with advances in medicine as they impact the care of those problems that are seen in an individual clinical work. Trainees and faculty, who mostly are inspired to provide compassionate, high-quality clinical care, feel empowered by EBM to critique the literature with respect to its helpfulness as a tool for clinical problem solving. Trainees and faculty read the abstract (to get the question), examine the methods to abstract the sampling frame, check the methods for validity, and look at the results section to find out what happened. This information is then vetted through clinical experience to make the best possible decision regarding the care of the patient. In a reversal of the usual course of things, research faculty sometimes find themselves in the odd position of restraining trainees from being too critical regarding study methods. As researchers ourselves, we plead that clinical research is hard to do and minor flaws do not necessarily invalidate clear and substantial outcomes.

What is evidence-based medicine?

The general approach to EBM involves the following steps: (1) construct a relevant, answerable question from a clinical case; (2) plan and carry out a search of the clinical literature; (3) critically appraise the literature for validity and usefulness; (4) apply the results of this appraisal to the clinical care of your patient; and (5) evaluate the outcome and use this information to frame new questions. In a probabilistic sense, applying the tools of EBM is similar to an insurance actuary assessing a client for automobile insurance. Actuaries calculate risk based on a number of factors such as driving records, sex, age, and so forth. Calculating these probabilities allows them to tell their companies how much to charge to make a profit. EBM allows the clinician to calculate the odds that certain interventions or tests will or will not help the patient based on empiric data and scientific principles. This information is then combined with clinical experience and the unique needs of the patient. Because EBM, strictly speaking, is not a mathematically driven algorithm that determines choices, but rather helps the clinician make better choices, it is not a threat to physicians' autonomy or to clinical nuances of the doctor–patient relationship.

Why evidence-based medicine in pediatric psychiatry?

Reintegrating psychiatry into medicine

Adopting the EBM approach to mental health education and practice reflects the reintegration of psychiatry into medicine as a whole [10]. During the period when psychoanalysis was preeminent in academic settings and in clinical practice, there was little support for medical models of mental illness or for empiric demonstration of the efficacy of treatments. This approach led to disengagement of psychiatry from the medical and scientific community. In the case of child psychiatry, this included little interaction with pediatrics or neurology. With advances spanning epidemiology, neuroscience, genetics, and empirically tested pharmacologic and psychosocial treatment of psychiatric disorders, the last 20 years has seen a sea change in the science of psychiatric illness in youth. Translation of these findings from academic settings into clinical practice remains a challenge. EBM provides a shared language and approach to the integration of science and clinical judgment that facilitates communication between psychiatric researchers and clinicians and with other medical specialties.

Evidence-based medicine eases the transition to a disease management approach

The three features of a disease management model—the concept of disease and diagnosis, the concept of etiology and treatment, and the nature of the doctor–patient relationship—come into play in pediatric psychiatry just as they do in the rest of medicine. For example, the treatment of pediatric obsessive-compulsive disorder (OCD) can be thought of as partially analogous to the treatment of juvenile-onset diabetes, with the caveat that the target organ (the brain, in the case of major mental illness) requires psychosocial interventions of much greater complexity. The treatment of diabetes and OCD involves medications (insulin for diabetes and a serotonin reuptake inhibitor for OCD) and an evidence-based psychosocial intervention that works, in part, by biasing the somatic substrate of the disorder toward more normal function. In diabetes, the psychosocial treatment of choice is diet and exercise; in OCD, it is cognitive behavioral therapy. Depending on the presence of risk and protective factors, not every patient has the same outcome. Bright youngsters from well-adjusted two-parent families typically do better with diabetes or OCD than those beset with tremendous psychosocial adversity. Thus, adversity, when present, appropriately becomes a target for intervention, usually to increase compliance with treatment of the primary illness. Finally, not everybody recovers completely, even with the best of available treatment, so some interventions need to target coping with residual symptoms such as diabetic foot care in diabetes and to help OCD patients and their families cope with residual symptoms skillfully.

Integrating psychiatry and psychology within a common framework

Given that many patients with psychiatric disorders receive drug and psychosocial interventions administered by mental health practitioners from different disciplines, there clearly is a need for a theoretic and practical framework for evaluating the effectiveness of diagnostic and treatment intervention that allows for a multidisciplinary team approach to mental health care. By way of example, the authors believe strongly that it is not possible to practice competent and ethical psychopharmacology without the availability of empirically supported psychotherapy. Similarly, it is not possible to practice competent and ethical psychotherapy without the availability of empirically supported psychopharmacology. Physicians (who typically write prescriptions) and psychologists (who, for the most part, have developed and typically are better versed in cognitive behavioral therapy) must join in the care of individual patients [11]. In this regard, the current generation of comparative treatment trials (eg, see the article by Jensen [12]) nicely models the benefits and the difficulties of multidisciplinary practice in which practitioners of both disciplines become stakeholders for the experiment (the research question) or the benefit of the individual patient (the clinical question). Without this commitment to multidisciplinary practice (which our experience shows is facilitated by EBM), we shortchange our patients.

Keeping up

Over the course of a clinician's professional life, a disparity frequently develops between clinical judgment and familiarity with current knowledge [1]. Increasing practice demands combined with often-outdated, traditional sources of information such as book chapters or pharmaceutic company–funded print materials perpetuate opinion-based decision making. It probably is true that 10 things account for 90% of the clinical activities in a clinical practice. For example, if patients with eating disorders are commonly seen in one's practice, keeping up with this clinical condition is mandatory; if not, keeping up is background reading, with the option (preferred) to refer those patients to someone for whom an eating disorder is on the top 10 list. No one can keep up with everything. By providing a strategy for the efficient retrieval and rapid appraisal of available information so as to obtain a best-practice outcome for patients seen in one's clinical practice, EBM therefore facilitates keeping up with literature where it matters most.

The practice of evidence-based medicine

Evidence-based medicine begins with an answerable clinical question

EBM begins with asking whether the clinical question in hand is about foreground or background knowledge. Background knowledge questions ask about conditions, illnesses, syndromes, patterns of disease, and pathophysiology. Examples of background knowledge questions are What is ADHD? and What is pharmagenomics and how is it different from pharmacogenetics? A beginning trainee might ask this type of question, which is best answered by using clinically oriented reviews in standard medical textbooks or journals to gain a general understanding of clinical issues. As with the art of medicine, background questions generally precede foreground questions, which seek specific information that is directly relevant to making decisions about patient care. An example of a foreground question is "In children and adolescents with OCD, does a selective serotonin reuptake inhibitor compared with placebo reduce the symptoms of OCD over 12 weeks of treatment"? Foreground questions are best answered by way of a critical appraisal of the scientific evidence base from the published literature. As shown in Table 1, the EBM approach to foreground questions depends on building an answerable clinical question. What makes a clinical question well built? First, the question should be directly relevant to the

Table 1
Framing an answerable question

Patient or problem	Intervention	Comparison intervention	Outcome
Description of the patient or the target disorder of interest	Could include: Exposure Diagnostic test Prognostic factor Therapy	Relevant most often when looking at therapy questions, but can include "gold standard" diagnostic test or expected untreated outcome	Clinical outcome of interest to you and your patient

problem at hand. Next, the question should be phrased to facilitate searching for a precise answer. To achieve these aims, the question must be focused and well articulated for all four parts of its "anatomy" [13]. In this regard, we typically frame foreground questions as a "PECO":

- What is the **population**?
- What is the **exposure**? (can be a diagnostic test or an active treatment)
- What is the **control or comparison** condition? (can be a "gold standard" test or a treatment)
- What is the desired **outcome**?

The following is an example of a treatment question framed as a PECO: In children with ADHD and Tourette's syndrome (the population), what is the effect of clonidine, methylphenidate, or combined clonidine and methylphenidate (the exposure) relative to placebo (the control) in reducing ADHD and tic symptoms over 6 weeks of treatment (the outcome)? After the question is formulated, the next step is to determine how to find the best evidence [14].

Searching the literature

To find the best evidence, we turn to on-line resources because they are readily available and provide timely information. (Because these resources are rapidly evolving, we consulted with the experienced staff at Duke Medical Library who provided the suggestions for the search resources that are listed in Boxes 1 and 2). A good starting point for a search is PubMed, which is easily accessible and comprehensive [9]. The Clinical Queries Service in PubMed uses well-developed filters that limit searches to specific research methodologies or systematic reviews and meta-analyses. The research methodology filters are divided into the categories of therapy, diagnosis, etiology, and prognosis, and users can designate searches to be sensitive or specific. These filters provide searches that are far more targeted than those obtained by typing "diagnosis" into the search engine.

To answer our previous PECO (What is the effect of clonidine, methylphenidate, or combined clonidine and methylphenidate in reducing ADHD and tic symptoms in children with ADHD and Tourette's syndrome?), we performed a search of Medline (through PubMed). By using the Clinical Queries Service,

---

Box 1. Searching for the evidence

Systems (comprehensive resources)

　　Clinical evidence (www.clinicalevidence.com)
　　Collections of evidence-based guidelines

Synopses (structured abstracts)

　　Evidence-Based Mental Health (http://ebmh.bmjjournals.com/)
　　American College of Physicians Journal Club (www.acpjc.org)

Syntheses (systematic reviews)

　　Cochrane Database
　　DARE (http://agatha.york.ac.uk/darehp.htm)

Studies (original research)

　　PubMed
　　OVID
　　PsychInfo

---

specifying a research methodology filter of therapy with an emphasis on specificity (to focus the inquiry), and using the search terms *ADHD* and *Tourette's*, we identified an 11-site randomized controlled trial done by the Tourette's Syndrome Study Group [15]. (These investigators concluded that clonidine or methylphenidate used alone and especially in combination is effective for ADHD disorder in children with tics.) In the absence of a well-constructed and executed empiric study, weaker evidence can (and should) be used if available but with less confidence regarding its applicability [7]. Because performing effective searches is a critical component of EBM, it is strongly recommended that readers refer to the book by Sackett et al [1] or the EBM tutorials, examples of which are listed in Box 2, for more complete details.

　　To the extent that the proliferation of EBM resources reflects a maturing scientific evidence base, is it possible (even in pediatric psychiatry) to find systematic reviews that make life easier for the busy clinician by summarizing existing literature in EBM format. These system reviews include comprehensive resources such as Clinical Evidence, structured abstracts as found in Evidence-Based Mental Health and the American College of Physicians Journal Club, and systematic reviews such as the Cochrane Database of Systematic Reviews (which is one of the four databases in the Cochrane Library). For example, a recent Cochrane review of tricyclic antidepressants concluded that these medications are not effective for major depression in children and adolescents [16]. OVID, a

Box 2. On-line resources

PubMed

The free on-line search engine that searches Medline, the National Library of Medicine's
Biomedical Database. Available at: www.pubmed.gov

PubMed tutorial

Well-designed modules for learning how to use PubMed. Pay special attention to MeSH headings, Boolean logic (ie, AND, OR), and the Clinical Queries Section. The link can be found at the PubMed site or at: www.nlm.nih.gov/bsd/pubmed_tutorial/m1001.html

OVID

Contains Medline, full-text articles, the Cochrane Library, and the ACP Journal Club www.acpjc.org). Available at: www.ovid.com

Clinical Evidence On-Line

Published by the *British Medical Journal* and a good source of current evidence. Doctors who are registered with United Health Foundation and who receive a copy in the mail have free access. You can sign up at www.unitedhealthfoundation.org. Available at: www.clinicalevidence.com

Tripdatabase

A metasearch engine that searches 61 EBM sites, including on-line journals such as the *British Medical Journal*, *Journal of the American Medical Association*, and *New England Journal of Medicine*. Also includes guidelines, electronic textbooks, and patient information leaflets. Available at: www.tripdatabase.com

National Guideline Clearing House

Produced by the US Department of Health and Human Services in association with other organizations. It contains evidence-based clinical practice guidelines and allows users to compare guidelines. Available at: www.guideline.gov

---

Evidence-Based Mental Health

Quarterly journal published by the *British Medical Journal*. Available at: ebmh.bmjjournals.com

EBM tutorials

SUNY Health Sciences EBM course
www.servers.medlib.hscbklyn.edu/ebm/toc.html
Duke EBM site: www.mclibrary.duke.edu/respub/guides/ebm
Duke/UNC EBM site: www.hsl.unc.edu/lm/ebm/index.htm

---

search engine that contains most of these databases, is available in many medical libraries or by subscription. Thus, as indicated in Box 3, which depicts the strength of the evidence for treatment outcome studies, the ideal search strategy begins with a systematic review (which requires multiple studies subjected to a meta-analysis), followed by single studies, and then the level of evidence for which less confidence is merited. The goal here is not to answer the question of whether there is evidence but to condition clinical recommendations on the strength of available evidence. When conclusive evidence is present (as in the tricyclic example), dogmatism regarding how to select among clinically reasonable choices is reasonable; when it is lacking, expert opinion and clinical experience occupy a more prominent place.

Evidence-based medicine as applied to diagnosis, therapy, harm, and prognosis

The care of the individual patient raises many questions. The process of evidence-based clinical practice involves the resolution of a searchable clinical

---

Box 3. A hierarchy of strength of evidence for treatment decisions

Systematic review of randomized trials
Single randomized trial
Systematic review of observational studies addressing patient-important outcomes
Single observational study addressing patient-important outcomes
Physiologic studies
Unsystematic clinical observations

Table 2
Four types of clinical questions framed in terms of population, exposure, comparison, and outcome (a PECO)

Clinical question	Clinical case	Population	Exposure/intervention	Comparison	Outcome
Diagnosis	10-y-old boy referred with recurrent sudden onset of eye blinking, cough, fine movements of his fingers, frequent hand washing and fear of germs	Prepubertal males with recurrent, abrupt onset tics, choreiform movements, compulsions and obsessions	Serial serum antistreptococcal antibody titer	Nasopharyngeal throat culture	Diagnosis of pediatric autoimmune neuropsychiatric disorder associated with strep
Treatment	8-y-old girl with recurrent sexual thoughts about boys and frequent hand washing and repetitive jumping up and down 5 times is referred for therapy	Prepubertal girls with obsessions and compulsions	Initial treatment with cognitive behavioral therapy	Treatment with supportive counseling	Clinically significant improvement of the obsessions and compulsions
Harm	Parent of a 12-y-old boy with ADHD wants to stop stimulants because he is afraid his son will become a substance abuser	Pubescent boys with ADHD	Cohort study of those taking stimulant medication	Cohort of ADHD boys not taking stimulant medication	Prevalence of substance abuse in ADHD boys taking stimulant medication compared to those who did not take stimulant medication
Prognosis	Parent wants to know if her 5-y-old daughter who is a picky eater will have an eating disorder as an adolescent	Preschool girls who are picky eaters	Cohort study of preschool girls who are picky eaters	Cohort of preschool girls who are not picky eaters	Prevalence of eating disorders in adolescent girls who were picky eaters as preschool children compared to adolescent girls without eating disorders who were not picky eaters as preschoolers

question. As indicated in Table 2, which provides examples of the four types of clinical questions and their PECOs, EBM addresses the four most common clinical questions [9]:

- Diagnosis involves establishing the power of a test to differentiate between those with and without a target condition or disease [17,18]. The diagnostic process involves the generation of possibilities and their associated likelihood ratios. A likelihood ratio for a given diagnostic test result provides the odds that that test result comes from a person who has the disease for which the test was ordered. When the likelihood ratio is multiplied by the "pretest" odds that your patient has the disease, the product is the "post-test" odds that the person has the disease. With a likelihood ratio nomogram for estimating post-test odds in hand, the clinician factors in his or her clinical expertise to select from among available test choices to avoid unnecessary testing, find the most likely test outcome, and rule out the most important outcomes that require treatment or are most responsive to treatment.
- Therapy involves determining the effect of different treatments on improving patient function or avoiding adverse events [19,20]. The answer to therapy questions is found in well-designed studies that have appropriately selected patients who are randomly assigned to a specified treatment or a control condition, treated, and assessed in their assigned groups regarding response status at the end of the study. The EBM statistic commonly used is the number needed to treat (NNT), which is defined as the number of patients who must receive a particular therapy for one patient to benefit. Mathematically, the NNT is the inverse of the absolute risk reduction or, for improvement, absolute benefit increase. For example, if 60% of subjects respond in the active treatment group and 40% in the placebo condition, the absolute benefit increase is 0.2 and the NNT is 5. You might tell a patient that an NNT of 5 means that the chance that he or she will benefit in this way from the treatment is 1 in 5. The analogous statistic for treatment-induced harm (an adverse event or outcome) is the number needed to harm, with the ratio of the NNT to the number needed to harm being the benefit/risk ratio.
- Harm/causation involves ascertaining the effects of potentially harmful agents on patient function, morbidity, and mortality [21]. In contrast to randomized treatment outcome studies in which the risk of harm is established against a control condition, harm in the sense of causation relies on observational studies in which personal choice or happenstance is the determinant for exposure or nonexposure to an agent. The EBM statistic used in harm/causation (from case control studies) is the odds ratio, defined as the ratio of the odds of being exposed in subjects with the target disorder divided by the odds in favor of being exposed in control subjects without the target disorder (ie, the ratio of the odds in exposed versus unexposed subjects).
- Prognosis involves estimating the future course of a patient's disease [22]. Knowledge about a patient's prognosis can help with the choice of whether

THE DUKE UNIVERSITY MODEL

to treat and what treatment to choose. Observational studies that select a particular group with features that may affect the prognosis are followed over time (exposure) to see whether they have the target outcome (disease or survival). Studies of disease prognosis typically employ survival curves, which graphically represent the number of events occurring over time or the chance of being free of these events over time.

Evidence-based medicine as applied to patient care guidelines

Within the EBM framework, guidelines are defined as systematically developed statements that assist practitioners and patients in making decisions about appropriate health care for specific clinical circumstances [23,24]. In contrast to unsystematic clinical reviews, which typically focus on a content area rather than on a specific clinical question or a set of questions linked to clinical decision nodes, a systematically assembled guideline (1) begins with a clear question (eg, what cognitive behavioral therapy components are effective as initial treatment for the depressed teenager) or a set of decision nodes (eg, specification of best-practice treatment for OCD in a stages of treatment model); (2) uses an explicit search strategy; (3) specifies criteria for evaluating the evidence; (4) provides a clear statement of real or potential biases in interpretation of the review; and (5) concludes with a recommendation for how to use the guideline in making decisions about the care of individual patients. As a result, an empirically based guideline framed in EBM terms provides expert consultation (without the expert) regarding best-practice options "at the bedside."

Applying the evidence to decisions about patient care

Whether for the care of individual patients or for decisions regarding systems issues such as specifying treatment options in a mental health center or managing a drug formulary, the essence of applying available evidence to patient care involves assessing the validity, clinical importance, and applicability of the evidence by asking the following questions: Can I trust this information? Is there a high or sufficient density of valid information to which I need to pay attention (eg, follow the recommendations in all or almost all cases)? If true, will the use of this information make an important difference in the care of my patients? Is this importance highlighted in the article I reviewed? Will the evidence translate to my patient care setting or to my patients' situation? Are there prognostic factors that increase or decrease the probability that my patients will follow the probabilities identified in the article? Does the article provide guidelines to the application of the evidence in implementing patient care? Given that I propose to use the recommendations in caring for my patients, how will I evaluate the outcome of this decision?

Teaching evidence-based medicine

Overview

The older paradigm of medical education, which has strong echoes in the American College of Graduate Medical Education requirement for child psychiatry training programs [25], emphasizes unsystematic observations from clinical practice, reasoning from basic principles of disease pathophysiology, traditional medical training with an emphasis on apprenticeship, and an emphasis on current content that often is derived from materials offered by pharmaceutic companies. In contrast, EBM provides a heuristically valuable philosophic framework for systematically integrating research into clinical practice that embraces clinical experience in the context of systematic rules for accessing and interpreting the best available evidence [1]. Not surprisingly, it is impossible to implement EBM at the patient level without knowledge of the *Diagnostic and Statistical Manual of Mental Disorders, Fourth Edition* and instruction in clinical interviewing skills, both of which form part of the foundational skills necessary for evidence-based practice. Hence, EBM, to some extent, is a higher-order skill that depends on prior clinical experience and good clinical practice, much of which is best encapsulated in background question readings and in direct clinical supervision.

Evidence-based medicine didactics

EBM can be taught effectively in multiple settings, although most programs that have successfully transitioned to EBM emphasize small group learning experiences in which didactic material is introduced, discussed, and practiced. Readily available textbooks provide valuable theory (eg, how to think probabilistically) and practical examples of EBM as applied to real-world clinical problems [1,2,7]. Worksheets (see Appendix A for a sample treatment worksheet) that facilitate critical appraisal of the literature on diagnosis, prognosis, treatment outcome, and other topics are widely available and make seminar preparation easier.

Evidence-based medicine at the bedside

One tool for bringing EBM directly to patient care in the teaching context is the EBM "prescription" [26]. An EBM prescription is a learning assignment cowritten by a supervisor and a student that describes the clinical problem that generated the question, defines the question in the form of a PECO, and identifies who is responsible for answering the question and over what time period (Fig. 1). Because everyone is always "too busy," an EBM prescription makes sure that patient care problems are pursued and teaching value is maximized. The result is to help students practice the important lifelong habit of using EBM on a daily basis to help answer clinical questions. Educational prescriptions can be included on rounds, at sign-out, during supervision, and during seminar and journal clubs. Prescriptions can be written by students for faculty and by faculty for students.

R$_x$ **Educational Prescription**

Patient's Name	Learner:

3-part Clinical Question

Target Disorder:

Intervention (+/- comparison):

Outcome:

Date and place to be filled:

Presentations will cover:
1. search strategy;
2. search results;
3. the validity of this evidence;
4. the importance of this valid evidence;
5. can this valid, important evidence be applied to your patient;
6. your evaluation of this process.

Fig. 1. Educational prescription.

When a willing librarian is present, an educational prescription is an ideal mechanism to teach enhanced search strategies that can help "fill" the prescription.

Critically appraised topic

One of the many practical by-products of evidence-based practice has been the development of CATs. After generating potential clinical inquiries in the PECO format and attempting to answer them with the best evidence available, the need to appraise the evidence for its validity and applicability becomes a necessary step before integrating that knowledge into practice. To this end, CATs, which use the EBM worksheet format, were invented by general medicine fellows at McMaster University as a method for honing their critical appraisal skills and improving their abilities to teach at the bedside. Because CATs are patient based, they allow clinicians at various stages of their careers to integrate their academic skills and clinical expertise in a way that applies directly to patient care. Although individual CATs may have potential limitations such as limited peer review, inferior evidence, single-investigation basis, and likelihood of obsolescence in the near future, generating them is a useful tool from educational and clinical decision-making standpoints. The therapy CAT (Appendix B), generated by Grace Thrall, MD, General Psychiatry Residency Training Director at Duke Medical Center, exemplifies this process. The software program CATMaker, published as shareware by the Center for Evidence Based Medicine http://www.cebm.net/catmaker.asp), greatly simplifies the generation of CATs by providing worksheet templates and performing the necessary calculations.

Library tools and on-line resources

As shown in Box 2, which lists readily available Internet-based instructional resources, the best friend that an EBM instructor can have is an EBM-oriented librarian. Librarians are especially skilled at demonstrating and providing hands-on practice with search strategies across the various levels of information represented in Box 1.

Evidence-based medicine gadgets

Given the tremendous growth in wireless and portable technology in recent years and the need for remote access to massive databases, it should be no surprise that EBM would makes its way into the world of personal digital assistants. Along with the ability to access the Internet, organize your schedule, or play a game of chess while waiting at the airport, these devices have opened a new level of portability to the accessibility and processing of digital information in the world of health care. Along with such applications as statistical software, medical calculators, textbooks, and drug references, a number of personal digital assistant software products are now available that allow inquisitive minds to access the latest clinical evidence and practice guidelines (Table 3). One recent addition to the list of clinically applicable software is PICOmaker. Available through the Uni-

Table 3
Examples of evidence-based applications for personal digital assistants

Category	Software	Resources
Calculators	MedCalc	Palmgear, www.palmgear.com
	EBM Calculator v1.2	University of Toronto Center for Evidence-Based Medicine, www.cebm.utoronto.ca
Web page interfaces	Avantgo	Avantgo (my.avantgo.com/home)
Textbooks	Harriet Lane Handbook	Mobipocket, www.mobipocket.com
	Harrison's Internal Medicine	Franklin Electronic Publishers, www.franklin.com
	DSM-IV TR	Franklin
	5-minute Pediatric Consult	Franklin
Recent literature review	InfoRetriever	InfoPoems, www.infopoems.com
	JournalToGo	JournalToGo, www.journaltogo.com
	Mobile MDConsult	MDConsult, www.mdconsult.com
	Ovid@Hand	OVID, www.ovid.com/site/products/ tools/ovidhand
Drug references	ePocrates Rx	ePocrates, www2.epocrates.com
	Tarascon Pocket Pharmacopoeia	Tarascon Publishing, www.tarascon.com
	Mobile Micromedex	Thomson Micromedex, www.micromedex.com
	PDR	Physicians' Desk Reference, www.pdr.net

versity of Alberta Library Web site, PICOmaker is a free palm-based application that allows users to create and store queries in the PECO/PICO (population, exposure/intervention, comparison, and outcome) format for later reference.

Faculty development

To bring EBM to the bedside in the context of training requires a program-level commitment to (1) teach EBM in formal didactic settings, (2) practice using EBM in the clinical settings in which training takes place, and (3) role model EBM on the part of faculty in supervision and in faculty practices. In contrast to departments of pediatrics or internal medicine in which EBM more often than not has become the standard heuristic, most faculty members in psychology and in psychiatry departments may not have been trained in or may not use EBM. To make the transition to EBM, faculty support is essential, for without active involvement of most of the faculty, the move from EBM didactics (requiring relatively few faculty) to EBM-oriented patient care in the clinic (requiring many more faculty) will be hindered. In addition to an orientation to the history and theory of EBM, this transition will be aided by specific instruction for faculty in formulating a question; searching the literature; using worksheets to CAT articles on diagnosis, prognosis, treatment, and harm/causation; and the use of the educational prescription as a teaching tool. As with teaching EBM to trainees, the learning process will be facilitated by small-group methods that encourage active participation of participants, hands-on practice with EBM tools, ready availability of EBM resources (including an EBM librarian and computer support services), and the support and encouragement from the department chair and child and adult training directors. Lastly, old habits tend to persist or, put differently, thinking probabilistically often does not come easily to faculty wedded to older models of teaching and clinical care. Nevertheless, it our experience that faculty who initially are reluctant to embrace EBM eventually become socialized by trainees (an enthusiastic chief resident is invaluable) who approach supervision using EBM language.

Related initiatives at Duke

Integrated child and adolescent residency program

In addition to becoming an essential core feature of the Duke general adult psychiatry training and the traditional child and adolescent training programs, EBM also has served as a bridge between the adult and child training programs. Due to the acute shortage of researchers in the field of child and adolescent psychiatry, there has been a national effort to foster and accelerate the entrance of medical students into research in the field. At Duke, this need was matched with a mutual recognition that a close collaboration between the adult general program and the child and adolescent program using the newly established platform of EBM would allow a comprehensive "dual-degree," 6-year clinical and research training program that would prepare residents for a career in academic child psychiatry research and board certification in adult psychiatry and in child and adolescent psychiatry. Linked by the shared principles of EBM, the program integrates research with clinical training and integrates child and adolescent clinical training with adult training. Research and child psychiatry training begin early and continue throughout residency. Trainees are assigned clinical and research faculty mentors in child psychiatry from their first postgraduate year onward. Trainees receive guidance in writing a career development award in the fifth or sixth postgraduate year. Early, intensive immersion in child psychiatry research during the first postgraduate year fosters early professional identity development as a child and adolescent psychiatry researcher. Sponsored research provides eligibility in the fifth and sixth years for the National Institutes of Health loan repayment program. If successful, the integrated child training program should help train the next generation of researchers in pediatric psychiatry.

Child and Adolescent Psychiatry Trials Network

It is widely acknowledged that the cultural shift toward evidence-based practice now underway in psychiatry [6,27] requires that research be seen as integral rather than separate from clinical practice [28]. It is less widely acknowledged that using high-quality research evidence to guide clinical practice has as many implications for researchers as it does for clinicians [29,30]. Although substantial progress has been made in developing and testing new treatments, researchers, for the most part, have failed to design trials that maximize clinical utility for practicing clinicians and other decision makers. Stated in terms of the contrary position, current best evidence often is not perceived by decision makers as relevant to clinical practice, thereby substantially diluting its impact [31]. To speed the translation of clinical research into medical practice, the National Institutes of Health has emphasized the need for practical clinical trials that are designed explicitly to aid decision makers in making decisions about patient care, whether this be at the doctor–patient or policy level [32]. In this context, Duke University and the American Academy of Child and Adolescent Psychiatry have joined together with National Institute of Mental Health funding to build a practical clinical trials network: the Child and Adolescent Psychiatry Trials Network (CAPTN; www.captn.org) [33]. Guided in the selection of specific questions by CAPTN members and expert advisory panels, CAPTN will focus on two critically important clinical issues: (1) obtaining randomized evidence regarding the effectiveness of widely used but understudied combined drug treatments; and (2) the short- and long-term safety of pharmacotherapy. Because the sole purpose of CAPTN is aiding decision makers in making decisions about patient care, CAPTN will go a long way toward increasing the evidence-base regarding practicable treatments and will disseminate EBM approaches further by presenting the results of CAPTN trials within an EBM framework. Furthermore, established practical clinical trials networks in other areas of medicine have been successful, in part, because the network participants were trained in network protocols during their fellowships and continued to participate in running protocols after entering private practice [34,35]. By emphasizing participation by trainees, CAPTN will bring EBM to the forefront not only with respect to accessing existing literature but also in generating that literature.

Summary

As applied to the training of child and adolescent psychiatrists in the Division of Child and Adolescent Psychiatry, Department of Psychiatry at Duke University Medical Center, EBM has become a well established and welcome heuristic platform for teaching residents (and faculty) how to integrate the best of evolving science with the art and wisdom of clinical medicine.

Appendix A. Example worksheet for evaluating a treatment study

Are the results of the study valid?

1. Was the assignment of patients to treatment randomized?
2. Were all patients who entered the trial properly accounted for and attributed at its conclusion? Was follow-up complete? Were patients analyzed in the groups to which they were randomized (intention to treat analysis)?

3. Were patients, their clinicians, and study personnel "blind" to treatment?
4. Were the groups similar at the start of the trial? Baseline prognostic factors (demographics, comorbidity, disease severity, other known confounders) balanced or adjusted for?
5. Aside from the experimental intervention, were the groups treated equally?

What were the results?

1. How large was the treatment effect? Absolute risk reduction? Relative risk reduction? Number needed to treat?
2. How precise was the estimate of the treatment effect (confidence intervals around number needed to treat)?

Will the results help me in caring for my patients?

1. Can the results be applied to my patient care? Were patients similar for demographics, severity, comorbidity and other prognostic factors? Is there a compelling reason why the results should not be applied?
2. Were all clinically important outcomes considered? Other endpoints?
3. Are the likely treatment benefits worth the potential harms and costs?
4. Are your patients' and your values and preferences satisfied by the regimen and its consequences?

Appendix B. Example of a CAT: lithium plus interpersonal therapy for adolescent bipolar disorder with substance abuse

Bottom line

This small RCT, with significant methodologic weaknesses, finds that lithium and interpersonal therapy may be more effective than interpersonal therapy alone in improving the overall social and psychiatric functioning of adolescents with bipolar disorder and comorbid substance dependence. Three patients would need to be treated with lithium and interpersonal therapy compared with interpersonal therapy alone over 6 weeks to have one additional patient respond to treatment (ie, achieve a Children's Global Assessment Scale [CGAS] of >65). Nevertheless, the strength of this evidence without further validation currently is insufficient to support with confidence the use of lithium plus interpersonal therapy as a recommended treatment for patients similar to this sample.

Background

The prevalence of bipolar disorder in adolescents is similar to that in adults. Although lithium is the traditional cornerstone of treatment for adult bipolar disorder, there are no double-blind placebo-controlled studies of lithium for bipolar disorder in children or adolescents. The psychopharmacologic treatment of juvenile bipolar disorder is remarkably understudied, and treatment often is based on studies of adults. Adolescent bipolar disorder often is accompanied by secondary substance dependence.

Search terms

Search terms included *bipolar disorder, lithium, adolescence,* and *substance use disorders.*

Clinical case/question

Is lithium plus interpersonal therapy an effective treatment for adolescent bipolar disorder with secondary substance dependence?

Reference

Geller B, Cooper TB, Sun K, Zimerman B, Frazier J, Williams M, et al. Double-blind and placebo-controlled study of lithium for adolescent bipolar disorders with secondary substance dependency. J Am Acad Child Adolesc Psychiatry 1998;37(2):171−8.

Methods

This National Institute of Drug Addiction−funded 6-week randomized, placebo-controlled, double-blind, parallel group study was designed to evaluate the efficacy of lithium for adolescent bipolar disorders with secondary substance dependence. Inclusion criteria included boys and girls 12 to 18 years old with a minimum 2-month history of comorbid *Diagnostic and Statistical Manual of Mental Disorders, Third Edition, Revised* substance-dependence disorder and bipolar disorder (I or II) or major-depressive disorder with at least one of the adolescent predictors of future bipolar disorder, which preceded the substance dependence. Exclusion criteria included pregnancy, IQ <75, schizophrenic disorders, major medical or neurologic disease, or psychotropic drug use during the prior 4 weeks. One hundred sixty patients recruited by way of newspaper advertisements were screened; 39 were invited for assessment. Twenty-five eligible postscreening outpatients (64% male, 100% Caucasian, mean age 16.3 years) were stratified by bipolar I disorder, bipolar II disorder, or mania versus manic-depressive disorder and predictors of future bipolar disease, and then randomized to lithium (Eskalith) or placebo. Thirteen patients were allocated to lithium, adjusted to achieve a maintenance serum level of 0.9 to 1.3 mEq/L. Twelve patients were allocated to matching placebo. In addition, all patients were seen twice weekly for assessments and received weekly interpersonal therapy modified for use with families. Primary outcomes were not specified at the outset of the study. At each visit, mood items from the Schedule for Affective Disorders and Schizophrenia for School-Aged Children (K-SADS), Adolescent Diagnostic interview, lithium side effects scale, pregnancy tests, and pill count were measured. Once weekly, a random serum lithium level and random urine drug screen were obtained.

Validity

Potential sources of bias or threats to the validity of this study included the following:

- Small sample size
- Lack of a clearly defined null hypothesis and predetermined primary outcome variables
- The short trial length may be insufficient for the measurement of meaningful long-term improvements in mood symptoms, substance use, and social/psychiatric function
- Design included concurrent treatment with interpersonal therapy plus twice weekly in-person contacts with study personnel, which biases the trial against finding an effect for lithium
- Potential confounding effect of ongoing substance use by study participants on treatment response

Blinding of all important groups and concealed randomization were asserted but not described by the investigators. Treatment groups were similar on known important prognostic factors, with the exception of more school dropouts in the placebo group. Good follow-up was present, and intention-to-treat analysis of 21 of 25 of those randomized, using last observation carried forward for dropouts, was performed. The groups were treated similarly outside of the intervention. Generalizability may be limited by the characteristics of the study population: patients were predominantly white, male outpatients with serious mood and substance use disorders.

Results

Outcome	Time to outcome	Expected event rate for lithium + interpersonal therapy	Control event rate for placebo + interpersonal therapy	Significance Test	Absolute risk reduction (95% confidence interval)	Number needed to treat (95% confidence interval)
CGAS >65 "Responders"	6 wk	6/13 (46.2%)	1/12 (8.3%)	$F = 4.59$ $P = 0.044$	0.378 (0.065– 0.691)	3 (1–15)

The percentage of random urine samples that had positive drug assays after week 3 was reduced from ~40% to ~10% in the lithium group, versus essentially no reduction in the placebo group ($P = 0.028$). No significant differences existed between lithium and placebo on K-SADS mood items or the SDD items by themselves.

There were no significant differences in random serum lithium levels drawn at weeks 3 to 6 between responders and nonresponders. For the intent-to-treat sample, the mean random serum lithium level was 0.98 ± 0.33 mEq/L.

Adverse effects

Significant differences in the Side Effects Scale scores were found between the active and placebo groups for thirst, polyuria, nausea, vomiting, and dizziness. Polyuria was found in five of the active subjects (41.7%) compared with no subjects in the placebo group, and a similar percentage was found for polydipsia.

Comments

The dose of lithium used in the study remains unproved. The serum lithium concentrations recommended in adults have been applied to children; however, this has not been studied.

References

[1] Sackett D, Richardson W, Rosenberg W, Haynes B. Evidence-based medicine. 2nd edition. London: Churchill Livingston; 2000.

[2] Gray G. Evidence-based psychiatry. Arlington (VA): American Psychiatric Publishing; 2004.

[3] Burns BJ. Children and evidence-based practice. Psychiatr Clin N Am 2003;26(4):955–70.

[4] Weisz JR, Jensen PS. Efficacy and effectiveness of child and adolescent psychotherapy and pharmacotherapy. Ment Health Serv Res 1999;1(3):125–57.

[5] Lohr KN. Rating the strength of scientific evidence: relevance for quality improvement programs. Int J Qual Health Care 2004;16(1):9–18.

[6] Geddes J, Carney S. Recent advances in evidence-based psychiatry. Can J Psychiatry 2001; 46(5):403–6.

[7] Guyatt G, Rennie D. Users' guides to the medical literature: essentials of evidence-based clinical practice. Chicago: AMA Press; 2002.

[8] Meehl P. Why I do not attend case conferences. In: Meehl P, editor. Psychodiagnosis: selected papers. Minneapolis (MN): University of Minnesota Press; 1973. p. 398.

[9] Guyatt GH, Haynes RB, Jaeschke RZ, Cook DJ, Green L, Naylor CD, et al. Users' guides to the medical literature: XXV. Evidence-based medicine: principles for applying the users' guides to patient care. Evidence-Based Medicine Working Group. JAMA 2000;284(10):1290–6.

[10] March J, Wells K. Combining medication and psychotherapy. In: Martin A, Scahill L, Charney DS, Leckman JF, editors. Pediatric psychopharmacology: principles and practice. London: Oxford University Press; 2003. p. 326–46.

[11] March J, Mulle K, Stallings P, Erhardt D, Conners C. Organizing an anxiety disorders clinic. In: March J, editor. Anxiety disorders in children and adolescents. New York: Guilford Press; 1995. p. 420–35.

[12] Jensen PS. Fact versus fancy concerning the multimodal treatment study for attention-deficit hyperactivity disorder. Can J Psychiatry 1999;44(10):975–80.

[13] Richardson WS, Wilson MC, Nishikawa J, Hayward RS. The well-built clinical question: a key to evidence-based decisions. ACP J Club 1995;123(3):A12–3.

[14] Haynes RB. Of studies, summaries, synopses, and systems: the "4S" evolution of services for finding current best evidence. Evid Based Ment Health 2001;4(2):37–9.

[15] Tourette's Syndrome Study Group. Treatment of ADHD in children with tics: a randomized controlled trial. Neurology 2002;58(4):527–36.

[16] Hazell P, O'Connell D, Heathcote D, Henry D. Tricyclic drugs for depression in children and adolescents. Cochrane Database Syst Rev 2002;(2):CD002317.

[17] Jaeschke R, Guyatt GH, Sackett DL. Users' guides to the medical literature. III. How to use an article about a diagnostic test. B. What are the results and will they help me in caring for my patients? The Evidence-Based Medicine Working Group. JAMA 1994;271(9):703–7.

[18] Jaeschke R, Guyatt G, Sackett DL. Users' guides to the medical literature. III. How to use an article about a diagnostic test. A. Are the results of the study valid? Evidence-Based Medicine Working Group. JAMA 1994;271(5):389–91.

[19] Guyatt GH, Sackett DL, Cook DJ. Users' guides to the medical literature. II. How to use an article about therapy or prevention. A. Are the results of the study valid? Evidence-Based Medicine Working Group. JAMA 1993;270(21):2598–601.

[20] Guyatt GH, Sackett DL, Cook DJ. Users' guides to the medical literature. II. How to use an article about therapy or prevention. B. What were the results and will they help me in caring for my patients? Evidence-Based Medicine Working Group. JAMA 1994;271(1):59–63.

[21] Levine M, Walter S, Lee H, Haines T, Holbrook A, Moyer V. Users' guides to the medical literature. IV. How to use an article about harm. Evidence-Based Medicine Working Group. JAMA 1994;271(20):1615–9.

[22] Laupacis A, Wells G, Richardson WS, Tugwell P. Users' guides to the medical literature. V. How to use an article about prognosis. Evidence-Based Medicine Working Group. JAMA 1994;272(3):234–7.

[23] Wilson MC, Hayward RS, Tunis SR, Bass EB, Guyatt G. Users' guides to the medical literature. VIII. How to use clinical practice guidelines. B. What are the recommendations and will they help you in caring for your patients? The Evidence-Based Medicine Working Group. JAMA 1995;274(20):1630–2.

[24] Hayward RS, Wilson MC, Tunis SR, Bass EB, Guyatt G. Users' guides to the medical literature. VIII. How to use clinical practice guidelines. A. Are the recommendations valid? The Evidence-Based Medicine Working Group. JAMA 1995;274(7):570–4.

[25] Sargent J, Sexson S, Cuffe S, Drell M, Dugan T, Ferren P, et al. Assessment of competency in child and adolescent psychiatry training. Academic Psychiatry 2004;28:18–26.

[26] Rucker L, Morrison E. The "EBM Rx": an initial experience with an evidence-based learning prescription. Acad Med 2000;75(5):527–8.

[27] Geddes J, Goodwin G. Bipolar disorder: clinical uncertainty, evidence-based medicine and large-scale randomised trials. Br J Psychiatry Suppl 2001;41:s191–4.

[28] Geddes J, Reynolds S, Streiner D, Szatmari P. Evidence based practice in mental health [editorial]. BMJ 1997;315(7121):1483–4.

[29] Hotopf M, Churchill R, Lewis G. Pragmatic randomised controlled trials in psychiatry. Br J Psychiatry 1999;175:217–23.

[30] Tunis SR, Stryer DB, Clancy CM. Practical clinical trials: increasing the value of clinical research for decision making in clinical and health policy. JAMA 2003;290(12):1624–32.

[31] Norquist GS, Magruder KM. Views from funding agencies. National Institute of Mental Health. Med Care 1998;36(9):1306–8.

[32] Zerhouni E. Medicine. The NIH roadmap. Science 2003;302(5642):63–72.

[33] March J, Silva S, Compton S, et al. The child and adolescent psychiatry trials network (CAPTN). J Am Acad Child Adolesc Psychiatry, in press.

[34] Califf RM, DeMets DL. Principles from clinical trials relevant to clinical practice: Part I. Circulation 2002;106(8):1015–21.

[35] Califf RM, DeMets DL. Principles from clinical trials relevant to clinical practice: Part II. Circulation 2002;106(9):1172–5.

ELSEVIER
SAUNDERS

Child Adolesc Psychiatric Clin N Am
14 (2005) 297–306

CHILD AND
ADOLESCENT
PSYCHIATRIC CLINICS
OF NORTH AMERICA

Promoting the Implementation of Practices that are Supported by Research: The National Implementing Evidence-Based Practice Project

William C. Torrey, MD[a,b,*], David W. Lynde, MSW, LICSW[b], Paul Gorman, EdD[b]

[a]West Central Behavioral Health, Dartmouth-Hitchcock, 2 Whipple Place, Lebanon, NH 03766, USA
[b]West Institute at the New Hampshire–Dartmouth Psychiatric Research Center,
Dartmouth Medical School, 2 Whipple Place, Lebanon, NH 03766, USA

When people seek health care, they want to be offered the services that are most likely to help them achieve their desired outcome. Innovations in health care, however, often are slow to be adopted widely in the routine service settings [1]. Slow dissemination can occur even when a practice has strong, well-publicized research support. Like the rest of health care [2,3], the field of mental health would like to speed up the process of bringing practices that have been shown to work to the people who need them [4–6].

The National Implementing Evidence-Based Practice Project (EBP Project) is a response to the recognition that many adults who experience schizophrenia and other severe mental illnesses do not have access to services that had been demonstrated to be effective [7]. Numerous recent reviews of the research evidence identify a core set of mental health practices that help people with severe mental illness to obtain the outcomes they desire, such as reduced symptoms and increased function and quality of life [7–12]. These effective practices, however, are not routinely available to most people with severe mental illnesses across the country [7,13].

The EBP Project's goals are to (1) create resources designed to facilitate the implementation of well-defined, research-supported practices in routine community mental health settings; (2) use the resources to implement the practices in a range of settings; and (3) learn from the experience, so as to be able to implement

This article was supported by a grant from the West Family Foundation.
* Corresponding author. West Central Behavioral Health, Dartmouth-Hitchcock, 2 Whipple Place, Lebanon, NH 03766.
E-mail address: william.c.torrey@dartmouth.edu (W.C. Torrey).

practices more efficiently [14]. This article reviews the conceptual foundations of the EBP Project and reflects on the authors' experience to date.

The National Implementing Evidence-Based Practice Project's start

In December 1998, the Robert Wood Johnson Foundation sponsored a panel composed of a number of different stakeholders in the field of mental health to discuss the large gap between what is known about service effectiveness and what routinely is offered in our mental health systems. This group identified six practices that currently are supported strongly by research: collaborative pharmacologic treatment [15], assertive community treatment [16], family psychoeducation [17], supported employment [18], illness management and recovery skills [19], and integrated dual disorders treatment for substance abuse and mental illness [20]. The group also proposed a demonstration project that would help the field learn more about the implementation of evidence-based practices (EBPs).

Following the meeting, the proposed implementation project gained momentum and became the EBP Project. The original plan envisioned three phases: (1) a development phase to create implementation packages for each EBP, (2) a pilot study phase to field-test the implementation packages and to modify them as needed, and (3) a larger, hypothesis-testing study to learn more about practice implementation. The project currently is in Phase II (Table 1).

Phase I

From the beginning, the EBP Project has recognized that EBPs are important to the extent that they help persons with severe mental illnesses to attain their desired goals. Implementing EBPs is worthwhile because multiple studies have demonstrated that these services can help consumers obtain outcomes such as increased independent housing, competitive employment, and quality of life and

Table 1
Phases of the National Implementing Evidence-Based Practice Project

Project phase	Time	Description
Preproject	Fall 1998	The project idea is initiated at a Robert Wood Johnson Foundation–sponsored meeting
Phase I	Fall 2000–Spring 2002	Teams of stakeholders design and create implementation packages
Phase II	Spring 2002–current time	Sites in eight states use the implementation packages to implement the EBPs
		Implementation monitors gather data about the implementations from all stakeholders in agencies and systems

decreased homelessness, hospitalization, symptoms, and substance use [15–20]. The commitment to helping consumers move ahead with their lives and pursue their individual goals rather than just to achieve clinical stability often is described as facilitating a "recovery" process [21–24]. Because the idea is to promote consumer access to effective treatments, it is expected that more practices will be added to the original six as the evidence base that supports additional services continues to grow [8].

Design of the implementation package

The design of the implementation package was based on a review of the implementation literature and the combined implementation experiences of many administrators, clinicians, family advocates, and services researchers [25]. For reasons outlined below, the project concluded that the implementation package should be (1) reasonably intensive, (2) focused on stage-wise change, and (3) sensitive to site-specific conditions.

Intensive intervention

Reviews of the research on practice change conclude that passive educational approaches such as dissemination of clinical practice guidelines and didactic educational meetings are ineffective and unlikely to result in practice change [26,27]. Some distinctly active interventions have been more effective. Interactive education meetings and workshops [28], educational outreach visits [29], and audit and feedback [30] have been shown to have an impact on targeted practice outcomes; however, as Oxman et al [31] concluded after their review of the literature, there are "no magic bullets" for changing provider behavior in health care.

The literature supports the idea that intensity of effort is related to success in studies of practice change [32,33]. For example, combining multiple strategies to overcome challenges is more likely to be effective than using only one intervention [26,27,34]. In addition, changing complex practice behavior, such as implementing a team-based EBP, requires a higher level of effort than is needed to affect a relatively simple change such as influencing a prescription choice [32,35].

These conclusions and the advice of experienced services researchers led to an implementation package design that was relatively intensive. The package expects that the implementation will take about a year and that it is more likely to succeed if the efforts of multiple stakeholders are aligned in support of a practice. Stakeholders who play essential roles in mental health care include (1) mental health authorities who create administrative rules and financial incentives, (2) mental health program leaders who set priorities and organize care, (3) mental health practitioners who provide direct care, and (4) consumers and families who create demand for specific mental health services [25]. The implementation packages have materials to address the needs of each of these stakeholder groups.

Staged intervention

Implementing a new practice in a routine mental health care setting entails promoting change in the behavior of groups of mental health care providers. Focus groups conducted in New Hampshire and Baltimore, Maryland with frontline providers indicated that clinicians must be convinced, then taught, and then supported in doing a new practice. Their comments were consistent with the thoughts of business theorists who advocate a stage-wise approach to behavior change. Adopters of innovations move through a process from awareness of the opportunity to change to selection, adoption, implementation, and finally, incorporation of the innovation in their routine daily behavior [36]. Efforts to promote change require different interventions, depending on the user's stage in this process. For example, a state-sponsored conference with dynamic speakers may work to make providers aware of and motivated to use an EBP, whereas a system of clinical supervision and reinforcing paperwork may be what is needed to get a desired practice into daily effective use. Finally, to keep the EBP going, a different strategy such as regular public recognition of clinicians who offer effective practice may be required. In short, change occurs in stages, so different parts of the implementation packages were designed to explicitly address motivation to change (why change?), enabling change (how to change), and reinforcing change (how to maintain and improve the gains).

Site-specific intervention tailoring

Social marketing concepts also informed the design. Social marketing involves identifying the behaviors to be changed, identifying the audience, identifying the barriers to change, reducing the barriers to change, and assessing results [37–39]. Customizing the message to meet the needs and interests of the target audience is an essential element of social marketing. Some research supports the importance of social marketing in promoting health care practice improvement. For example, academic detailing is more effective if it has a social marketing component [29].

Implementing sites vary in terms of their culture and immediate challenges, yet each has to perceive the EBP as an answer to its needs for the implementation to be successful. To communicate the EBP's relevance and to help overcome the site-specific barriers, the implementation package must include someone who knows the site well and can translate the practice to fit local circumstances. This feature was designed into the implementation package in the role of the trainer/consultant.

Creation of the implementation packages

After the basic implementation package framework was designed, a team of researchers, clinicians, program managers and administrators, consumers, and family members was assembled to create the specific content for each EBP. The teams organized their effort around a basic, three-staged change model aimed to predispose stakeholders to offer the EBPs, enable implementation, and guide planning for long-term practice sustainability. Review panels, also composed of different stakeholders, reviewed the materials developed by the six EBP teams to ensure consistency of presentation and attention to the various perspectives of the different constituencies.

Each implementation package consists of complementary teaching materials, training, and consultation. The training materials, referred to as an implementation resource kit, include a research review; information sheets on the practice for consumers, families, practitioners, and program leaders; an introductory video; a skills demonstration video; a workbook for practitioners and their clinical supervisors; a Web site with information; implementation tips; outcomes information; a practice fidelity scale; and a general organizational index. Documents oriented toward specific stakeholder groups were written by the stakeholders or in close collaboration with them.

In addition to the implementation resource kit, the implementation packages include the provision of complementary training activities and consultation. The basic goal of the training is to help motivate administrators and practitioners to offer the practice and then to develop the necessary skills to provide the practice well. The goal of the year-long consultation is to assist the agency in evaluating and modifying polices and procedures to facilitate the implementation of the practice. The trainer/consultant works closely with the site implementation leader to train the staff, model effective clinical supervision on the EBP, and reconfigure the flow of daily work so that it supports the desired practice. The trainer/consultant also works with agencies to explore what consumer outcomes can be developed or used to provide feedback on practice effectiveness as a means to reinforce and constantly evaluate the practice.

Phase II

Phase II of the EBP Project currently is underway. The phase has multiple aims: (1) field-testing the different implementation packages in multiple sites in several states to see whether they succeed in facilitating high-fidelity practice implementation, (2) using the practical feedback from the experience to improve the implementation packages, (3) developing recommendations for implementing EBPs for state mental health authorities and implementing agencies, and (4) contributing to the assessment methodology for the future study of implementation process.

Eight states are participating in this phase. Each state agreed to develop a site selection process to obtain three to five agencies per practice. Implementing states also were responsible for securing a local trainer/consultant for each practice. In addition, states hired implementation monitors to gather qualitative information from a variety of stakeholders during the implementation process and for 1 year thereafter. Each state also agreed to reassess their policies and funding mechanisms based on feedback from pilot sites. Table 2 lists the states and the practices for phase II of the EBP Project.

Table 2
States and evidence-based practices for phase II of the National Implementing Evidence-Based
Practice Project

State	Evidence-based practices
Indiana	Assertive Community Treatment
	Integrated Dual Disorders Treatment
Kansas	Integrated Dual Disorders Treatment
	Supported Employment
Maryland	Family Psychoeducation
	Supported Employment
New Hampshire	Family Psychoeducation
	Illness Management and Recovery
New York	Assertive Community Treatment
	Illness Management and Recovery
Ohio	Integrated Dual Disorders Treatment
	Illness Management and Recovery
Oregon	Supported Employment
Vermont	Family Psychoeducation
	Illness Management and Recovery

Phase II has an evaluation component that includes on-site observation of the EBP implementation at all sites by implementation monitors who are not part of the implementation, computerized surveys of implementers, and focus groups with all stakeholders. These data now are being collected and organized for later analysis.

Early reflections on the phase II experience

Although data from the EBP Project are still being gathered and no formal analyses have been completed, the following sections highlight some general observations that may be made regarding the implementation progress so far with the set of current EBPs. These reflections flow from the feedback of trainer/consultants who are involved with the project in all of the states.

Implementing evidence-based practices is not a top priority for many

Although the mental health services research literature [6] and the President's New Freedom Commission on Mental Health report [13] have noted the chasm between the services that could be offered and the services that are offered to the people we serve, the impassioned call for radical improvement has not penetrated many state and local systems. The EBP Project's experience is that the culture at many practice sites is not naturally oriented toward thinking scientifically so that the sites are not always predisposed toward offering research-supported services. Likewise, state systems of care vary widely in their baseline commitment to building and maintaining an infrastructure to promote science-based services. Each state and site must find a strong clear response to the question, "why should we implement"? before it can actively engage in meeting the challenge of how to implement.

Practices that solve clear problems attract interest

As other implementers have found [40], practices that were perceived to meet a previously identified system need were easier to promote than those that were just seen as a good idea. When systems already knew that they wanted to enhance employment, they were eager to embrace Supported Employment; when systems saw that they needed more intensive outreach services to help people who were repeatedly hospitalized and had money earmarked for the task, they were glad for help in implementing Assertive Community Treatment; and when systems already knew that they were not effectively serving a large population of dually diagnosed people, they quickly moved into Integrated Dual Disorders Implementation. In contrast, Integrated Dual Disorders Treatment was hard to promote in other settings in which substance abuse was under-recognized and, therefore, not seen as a major obstacle to recovery.

Implementing an evidence-based practice is a complex project

Some investigators have drawn distinctions between simple, complicated, and complex problems to illustrate the nature of complex problems [41,42]. A simple problem (ie, baking a cake) is one that can be addressed effectively with a recipe that can be followed by a nonexpert, whereas a complicated problem (ie, sending off a rocket) requires the application of detailed expert knowledge. In contrast, complex problems (ie, raising a child) do not lend themselves to formulaic solutions, although past experience and the advise of experts sometimes can help. Succeeding in addressing one complex problem does not guarantee success on future, similar attempts.

Implementing an EBP is complex. Implementation often involves addressing numerous interconnecting challenges, from philosophy of care to finance to daily operations to personnel issues. In the EPB Project, for example, some sites did not begin with a recovery-oriented philosophy of treatment. Without an internalized commitment to consumer recovery, practitioners found it difficult to understand the benefits of competitive employment for people with serve mental illness or the hope and achievement of dual recovery for people with co-occurring disorders. The initial work of implementing at these sites required stepping back and facilitating a philosophic shift. Then, when sites became convinced that they wanted to implement the EBP, they were faced with redesigning the flow of daily work so that it supported the new practice. The task often involves getting professionals to provide service in a new, more structured manner, realigning financial resources, and configuring clinical operations to support the practice. These changes do not lend themselves to recipe or expert-dictated solutions but must be addressed with real people practicing under specific conditions. Each site requires a unique solution.

Leadership is essential

Because there does not appear to be any one formula for implementing an EBP, leaders must actively lead to get the implementation to occur. EBPs do not self-implement. Leadership includes articulating how the EBP fosters the mission of the agency or system and making the vision a reality through focused, committed change efforts over time. Leaders have many choices in how they can address the implementation challenges, and successful leaders seek specific approaches that flow from their intimate knowledge of their site's specific needs [43].

The role of trainer/consultant is critical and challenging

The implementation package includes on-site training and year-long consulting by a trainer/consultant to help the program leader tailor the practice to the site and the site to the practice. What makes the practices evidence based is that they contain generalizable knowledge that can bring benefit to consumers who seek help at sites beyond where the practice was developed and tested. To achieve that promise, the practice must be translated from the general back to the specific at the implementing sites [44]. The process is analogous, although more complex, to a physician applying generalizable medical knowledge to treat an individual patient. Like the physician, the effective trainer/consultant must have a very good grasp of the practice to be implemented and have the ability to help apply that knowledge in particular cases. In addition, like patients receiving help from physicians, implementing sites are more likely to follow the trainer/consultant's recommendations when he or she projects competence and confidence. Recruiting, training, and supporting these key individuals takes sustained effort at the mental health authority level.

Summary

Improving access to EBPs offers opportunities for all stakeholders in mental health. Consumers and families benefit from services that have proved their effectiveness in helping consumers to achieve goals that are meaningful to them. Offering effective practices is professionally fulfilling to practitioners who can see the contribution that their work is making to the recovery of the patients they serve. Public and agency mental health administrators benefit from being able to provide a higher degree of assurance that increasingly scarce mental health funds are being used to provide services that are effective in fulfilling their mission.

The EBP Project is seeking to learn how to efficiently promote and facilitate the implementation of EBPs. So far, the project has not uncovered any simple, generally applicable recipe for enabling practice change. Careful analysis of the extensive data currently being collected will provide important information for all stakeholders engaged in EBP implementation.

References

[1] Berwick DM. Disseminating innovations in health care. JAMA 2003;289(15):1969–75.
[2] Batalden PB, Stoltz PK. A framework for the continual improvement of health care: building and applying professional and improvement knowledge to test changes in daily work. Joint Commission Journal on Quality Improvement 1993;19(10):424–45.
[3] Committee on Quality Healthcare in America. Institute of Medicine: crossing the quality chasm: a new health system for the 21st century. Washington DC: National Academy Press; 2001.
[4] National Advisory Mental Health Council's Clinical Treatment and Services Research Workgroup. Bridging science and service. National Institutes of Health, 1999. Available at: www.nimh.nih.gov/publicat/nimhbridge.pdf. Accessed December 8, 2004.
[5] National Advisory Mental Health Council's Clinical Treatment and Services Research Workgroup. Translating behavioral science into action, 2000. Available at: www.nimh.nih.gov/publicat/nimhtranslating.pdf. Accessed December 8, 2004.
[6] Goldman HH, Ganju V, Drake RE, Gorman PG, Hogan M, Hyde PS, et al. Policy implications for implementing evidence-based practices. Psychiatr Serv 2001;52:1591–7.
[7] US Department of Health and Human Services. Mental health: a report of the Surgeon General. Rockville (MD): US Department of Health and Human Services, Substance Abuse and Mental Health Services Administration, Center for Mental Health Services, National Institutes of Health, National Institute of Mental Health; 1999.
[8] Drake RE, Goldman HH, Leff HS, Lehman AF, Dixon L, Mueser KT, et al. Implementing evidence-based practices in routine mental health settings. Psychiatr Serv 2001;52:179–82.
[9] Fenton W, Schooler N. Editors' introduction: evidence-based psychosocial treatment for schizophrenia. Schizophr Bull 2000;26:1–3.
[10] Kane JM. Pharmacologic treatment of schizophrenia. Biol Psychiatry 1999;46(10):1396–408.
[11] Lehman AF, Steinwachs DM, the Survey Co-Investigators of the PORT Project. Translating research into practice: the Schizophrenia Patient Outcomes Research Team (PORT) treatment recommendations. Schizophr Bull 1998;24:1–10.
[12] Miller AL, Chiles JA, Chiles JK, Crismon ML, Rush AJ, Shon SP. The Texas Medication Algorithm Project (TMAP) schizophrenia algorithms. J Clin Psychiatry 1999;60:649–57.
[13] New Freedom Commission on Mental Health. Achieving the promise: transforming mental health care in America. Final report. Rockville (MD): US Department of Health and Human Services; 2003 [Publication No. SMA-03–3832].
[14] Mueser KT, Torrey WC, Lynde D, Singer P, Drake RE. Implementing evidence-based practices for people with severe mental illness. Behav Mod 2003;27(3):387–411.
[15] Mellman TA, Miller AL, Weissman EM, Crismon ML, Essock SM, Marder SR. Evidence-based pharmacologic treatment for people with severe mental illness: a focus on guidelines and algorithms. Psychiatr Serv 2001;52(5):619–25.
[16] Phillips SD, Burns BJ, Edgar ER, Mueser KT, Linkins KW, Rosenheck RA, et al. Moving assertive community treatment into standard practice. Psychiatr Serv 2001;52(6):771–9.
[17] Dixon L, McFarlane WR, Lefley H, Lucksted A, Cohen M, Falloon I, et al. Evidence-based practices for services to families of people with psychiatric disabilities. Psychiatr Serv 2001;52: 903–10.
[18] Bond GR, Becker DR, Drake RE, Rapp CA, Meisler N, Lehman AF, et al. Implementing supported employment as an evidence-based practice. Psychiatr Serv 2001;52(3):313–22.
[19] Mueser KT, Corrigan PW, Hilton DW, Tanzman B, Schaub A, Gingerich S, et al. Illness management and recovery: a review of the research. Psychiatr Serv 2002;53:1272–84.
[20] Drake RE, Essock SM, Shaner A, Carey KB, Minkoff K, Kola L, et al. Implementing dual diagnosis services for clients with severe mental illness. Psychiatr Serv 2001;52:469–76.
[21] Anthony WA. Recovery from mental illness: the guiding vision of the mental health service system in the 1990s. Psychosocial Rehab J 1993;16:11–23.
[22] Anthony WA. A recovery-oriented service system: setting some system level standards. J Psychiatr Rehab 2000;24:159–68.

[23] Mead S, Copeland ME. What recovery means to us: consumers' perspectives. Community Ment Health J 2000;36:315–28.

[24] Torrey WC, Wyzik PF. The recovery vision as a service improvement guide for community mental health center providers. Community Ment Health J 2000;36(2):209–16.

[25] Torrey WC, Drake RE, Dixon L, Burns BJ, Flynn L, Rush AJ, et al. Implementing evidence-based practices for persons with severe mental illnesses. Psychiatr Serv 2001;52:45–50.

[26] Bero LA, Grilli R, Grimshaw JM, Harvey E, Oxman AD, Thomsom MA. Getting research findings into practice: closing the gap between research and practice: an overview of systematic reviews of interventions to promote the implementation of research findings. BMJ 1998;317:465–8.

[27] Grimshaw JM, Shirran L, Thomas R, Mowatt G, Fraser C, Bero L, et al. Changing provider behavior: an overview of systematic reviews of interventions. Med Care 2001;39(8):II-2–45.

[28] Thomson O'Brien MA, Freemantle N, Oxman AD, Wolf F, Davis DA, Herrin J. Continuing education meetings and workshops: effects on professional practice and health care outcomes (Cochrane Review). In: The Chochrane Library, Issue 4, 2002. Oxford: Update Software.

[29] Thomson O'Brien MA, Oxman DA, Haynes RB, Freemantle N, Harvey EL. Educational outreach visits: effects on professional practice and health care outcomes (Cochrane Review). In: The Cochrane Library, Issue 4, 2002. Oxford: Update Software.

[30] Thomson O'Brien MA, Oxman AD, Davis DA, Haynes RB, Freemantle N, et al. Audit and feedback: effects on professional practice and healthcare outcomes (Cochrane Review). In: The Chochrane Library, Issue 4, 2002. Oxford: Update Software.

[31] Oxman AD, Thomson MA, Davis DA. No magic bullets: a systematic review of 102 trials of interventions to improve professional practice. Can Med Assoc J 1995;153(10):1423–31.

[32] Davis DA, Thompson MA, Oxman AD, Haynes B. Evidence for the effectiveness of CME: a review of 50 randomized controlled trials. JAMA 1992;26:1111–7.

[33] Schulberg HC, Katon W, Simon GE, Rush AJ. Treating major depression in primary care practice: an update of the Agency for Health Care Policy and Research practice guidelines. ArchGen Psychiatr 1998;55:1121–7.

[34] Grimshaw JM, Russell IT. Effect of clinical guidelines of medical practice: a systematic review of rigorous evaluations. Lancet 1993;342:1317–22.

[35] Rogers EM. The challenge: lessons for guidelines from the diffusion of innovations. J Qual Improv 1995;21:324–8.

[36] Klein KJ, Sorra JS. The challenge of innovation implementation. Acad Manage Rev 1996;21(4):1055–80.

[37] Andreasen AR. Marketing social change: changing behavior to promote health, social development, and the environment. San Francisco (CA): Jossey-Bass; 1995.

[38] Lefebvre RC, Flora JA. Social marketing and public health intervention. Health Educ Q 1988;15(3):299–315.

[39] Walsh DC, Rudd RE, Moeykens BA, Moloney TW. Social marketing for public health. Health Aff 1993;12:104–19.

[40] Liberman RP, Eckman TA. Dissemination of skills training modules to psychiatric facilities: overcoming obstacles to the utilization of a rehabilitation innovation. Br J Psychiatr 1989;155(Suppl 5):117–22.

[41] Glouberman S, Zimmerman BJ. Complicated and complex systems: what would successful reform of Medicare look like? Discussion paper #8, Commission on the Future of Health Care in Canada. July, 2002.

[42] Plsek, P. Complexity and the adoption of innovation in health care. Accelerating quality improvement in health care: strategies to speed the diffusion of evidence-based innovations. A conference sponsored by the National Institute for Health Care Management Foundation and National Committee for Quality Health Care. January 27–28, 2003.

[43] Torrey WC, Finnerty M, Evans A, Wyzik P. Strategies for leading the implementation of evidence-based practices. Psychiatr Clin N Am 2003;26:883–97.

[44] Batalden P. When improvement doesn't happen as planned. Presentation for the New Hampshire–Dartmouth Psychiatric Research Center. Lebanon, NH. February 24, 2004.

ELSEVIER
SAUNDERS

Child Adolesc Psychiatric Clin N Am
14 (2005) 307–327

CHILD AND
ADOLESCENT
PSYCHIATRIC CLINICS
OF NORTH AMERICA

Federal, State, and Foundation Initiatives Around Evidence-Based Practices for Child and Adolescent Mental Health

David A. Chambers, PhD[a,*], Heather Ringeisen, PhD[a],
Enith E. Hickman, MPH[b]

[a]National Institute of Mental Health, National Institutes of Health, MSC 9631,
6001 Executive Boulevard, Bethesda, MD 20892-9631, USA
[b]Department of Health and Human Services, Centers for Medicare & Medicaid Services,
7500 Security Boulevard, Baltimore, MD 21244, USA

This article is a survey of many of the initiatives developed by federal and state agencies and foundations that focus on evidence-based mental health practices for children and adolescents. Although this is not an exhaustive summary of every initiative at national, state, and foundation levels, the article intends to show the tremendous interest in the development, dissemination, and implementation of evidence-based practice (EBP) in child and adolescent mental health that is held by various agencies and organizations. After a review of specific initiatives, several "next steps" for the field are suggested that might be developed in a subsequent series of initiatives. These steps include a better understanding of dissemination and implementation processes, increased clarity around definitions and terms, increased efforts to build infrastructure and support policy change, and the potential for an aggregation of data already gathered on the implementation of EBPs.

The last two decades have seen tremendous growth in our knowledge about how best to identify and treat behavioral and emotional disorders of childhood [1]. Although the knowledge base is admittedly far from complete, public demands for improved mental health services have pressed forward a discussion about the role of "evidence-based" interventions in everyday clinical practice.

The summary of initiatives and discussions represented in this article are from the perspectives of the authors. They do not necessarily represent the views of the US Department of Health and Human Services, the National Institute of Mental Health, Columbia University, or the New York State Office of Mental Health.
    * Corresponding author.
    E-mail address: dchambers@mail.nih.gov (D.A. Chambers).

Table 1
Resources for evidence-based mental health initiatives

Agency	Office/Initiative	Focus
Federal government		
Administration for Children and Families (ACF) http://www.acf.hhs.gov	Child Outcomes Research and Evaluation http://www.acf.hhs.gov/programs/core/index.html	Research activities and funding opportunities focusing on 4 bureaus of ACF
	Family and Child Experiences Survey (FACES) http://www.acf.hhs.gov/programs/core/ongoing_research/faces/faces_intro.html	Information on FACES study (Head Start)
Department of Education (DOE) http://www.ed.gov	Research and Training Center on Early Childhood Development http://researchtopractice.info	Translating knowledge into effective strategies for young children's success
	National Center for Evidence Based Practices for Students with Intensive Social, Emotional, and Behavioral Needs http://www.lehigh.edu/projectreach	Research on elementary/middle and secondary school children with intensive social, emotional, and behavioral needs
	The Center for Evidence-Based Practice: Young Children with Challenging Behavior http://challengingbehavior.fmhi.usf.edu/index.html	Interventions, information and research on young children with, or at risk for, behavioral problems
	Technical Assistance Center on Positive Behavioral Interventions and Supports (PBIS) http://www.pbis.org/english/	Dissemination and demonstrations of behavioral interventions
	Office of Special Education Programs and Projects (OSEP) http://www.ed.gov/about/offices/list/osers/osep/programs.html	Information on programs and projects supported by OSEP
Health Resources and Services Administration (HRSA) http://www.hrsa.gov	UCLA School Mental Health Project http://smhp.psych.ucla.edu	Addresses mental health and psychosocial concerns through school-based interventions
	Center for School Mental Health Assistance http://www.umaryland.edu	Expansion of mental health in schools
National Institute of Child Health and Human Development (NICHD) http://www.nichd.nih.gov	Interagency Education Research Initiative http://drdc.uchicago.edu/about/drdc_ieri.html	Evidence-based interventions for educational success

National Institute of Mental Health (NIMH) http://www.nimh.nih.gov	Services Research and Clinical Epidemiology Branch http://www.nimh.nih.gov/srceb/index.cfm	Supports research and intervention on organization, delivery, and financing of mental health services
	"Dissemination and Implementation Research in Mental Health" http:///grants.nih.gov/grants/guide/pa-files/PA-02-131.html	Program announcement
	"Practice, Effectiveness and Implementation Research within CMHS' Children's Service Sites" http://grants.nih.gov/grants/guide/pa-files/PA-04-019.html	Program announcement
	"Child and Adolescent Interdisciplinary Research Networks" http://grants1.nih.gov/grants/guide/rfa-files/RFA-MH-02-011.html	Request for Application (no longer active announcement)
	Services Research and Clinical Epidemiology Branch Conferences http://www.nimh.nih.gov/srceb/confs.cfm	Links to past and current conferences
Office of Juvenile Justice and Delinquency Prevention (OJJDP) http://ojjdp.ncjrs.org/	Blueprints http://www.colorado.edu/cspv/blueprints/index.html	Identification of effective violence prevention programs
	Mental Health and Juvenile Justice: Building a Model for Effective Service Delivery http://www.ncmhjj.com/projects/ojjdp.asp	Mental health needs of youth in juvenile justice system
Substance Abuse and Mental Health Services Administration (SAMHSA) http://www.samhsa.gov	Center for Mental Health Services http://www.samhsa.gov/centers/cmhs/cmhs.html	Agency's center for treatment and support services for mental health
	Safe Schools/Healthy Students http://www.mentalhealth.org/safeschools/	School violence reduction
	Systems of Care http://www.systemsofcare.net	Information and resources for the system of care approach
	National Child Traumatic Stress Network (NCTSN) http://www.ntcsnet.org	Research and interventions on child traumatic stress
	National Registry of Effective Practices http://modelprograms.samhsa.gov	Resource of evidence-based treatments for substance abuse and mental health
	Targeted Capacity Expansion grant announcement http://www.samhsa.gov/grants/content/2002/pa03001.htm	Grant announcement

(continued on next page)

Table 1 (*continued*)

Foundation	Initiative	Focus
Foundations		
Annenberg Foundation Trust at Sunnylands http://www.sunnylands.org	Adolescent Mental Health Initiative http://www.sunnylands.org/AMHI/	Disorders prevalent in adolescence
Annie E. Casey http://www.aecf.org	BlueSky Project (no website as of yet)	Linking 3 EBPs for antisocial and delinquent youth: FFT, MST, TFC
Commonwealth Fund http://www.cmwf.org	Healthy Steps for Young Children http://www.healthysteps.org	Health care practices for first three years of life, including behavioral and developmental issues
	Assuring Better Child Health and Development http://www.cmwf.org/programs/child/abcd_2ndpg.asp	Child development services for low-income children
	Pediatric Development and Behavior http://www.dbpeds.org	Funds supports development of web-based resource for developmental and behavioral screening
Robert Wood Johnson Foundation http://www.rwjf.org	Reclaiming Futures http://www.reclaimingfutures.org/	Teenagers involved in drugs, alcohol, and crime
	Center for Health and Health Care in Schools http://www.healthinschools.org/home.asp	Health service programs in schools, including mental health
	Free to Grow http://www.freetogrow.org	Head Start partnerships for prevention of substance abuse and child abuse

Agency		Focus
Kellogg Foundation http://www.wkkf.org/default.aspx	Ongoing Mental Health Funds	Foundation home page
Klingenstein Foundation http://www.ktgf.org/	Ongoing Mental Health Funds	Links between schools and mental health
John D. and Catherine T. MacArthur Foundation http://www.macarthur.org	Youth Mental Health Network	Clinic treatments and clinic systems effectiveness and implementation
State governments		
New York http://www.omh.state.ny.us/omhweb/ebp/children.htm		Evidence-based practices for children and families
Michigan http://www.michigan.gov/mdch/0,1607,7-132-2941_4868_7145- -,00.html		Child and adolescent mental health home page
Hawaii http://www.state.hi.us/doh/camhd/index.html		Child and adolescent mental health home page

The scientific community also has called for increased attention to bridging the gap between the current scientific state and ongoing clinical activities [2]. Finally, these issues have been placed at the forefront of multiple national publications on children's mental health. The New Freedom Commission Report [3], the report of the surgeon general's conference on children's mental health [4], and the National Institute of Mental Health (NIMH) "Blueprint for Change" report [5] clearly articulate the need to expand the use of EBPs within communities and increase the knowledge base about how this can be done. In response to these concerns, federal, foundation, and state agencies each have organized a series of initiatives that focus on program development, implementation, research endeavors, or policy change.

Within this article we review recent initiatives conducted by federal, foundation, and state organizations to promote the integration of evidence-based mental health interventions for children into routine clinical practice. (Please see footnote at beginning of article.) The initiatives described within this article do not represent an exhaustive summary but are meant to highlight the diverse and mounting array of activities in this area. Additional resources (including Internet addresses) for these initiatives and others are included in Table 1.

Federal activities

Several federal government agencies have organized initiatives to facilitate the integration of EBPs for children's mental health into real-world service delivery settings. Representative agencies within the US Department of Health and Human Services, US Department of Education, and US Department of Justice have launched independent programs and collaborative efforts to improve the quality of mental health services for children and adolescents.

National Institute of Mental Health

The NIMH is the primary agency within the National Institutes of Health responsible for conducting and supporting research to reduce the burden of mental illness. Over the last several years, NIMH has organized several activities to advance research on dissemination and implementation processes. These activities are intended to broaden our scientific understanding of how to move scientifically supported mental health interventions into community practice settings. Within this section, we describe five primary initiatives focused either in part or solely on children and adolescents: (1) interdisciplinary scientific networks, (2) state planning grants, (3) a dissemination and implementation research program announcement, (4) a call for research within the Center for Mental Health Services children's service sites, and (5) annual conferences related to issues in mental health services research.

In 2001, NIMH issued a request for applications for the development of interdisciplinary networks to foster innovative approaches to research in child and adolescent mental health. Applications were sought in several areas; one area focused on the dissemination and implementation of EBPs for child and adolescent mental health. The request for applications encouraged networks to include scientists from a diverse array of disciplines (eg, psychology, anthropology, organizational development, and marketing) along with representatives of key stakeholder groups to conceptualize frameworks for dissemination or implementation research. Three dissemination and implementation networks received funding for a 3-year period; one network focuses on autism and telemedicine, another on child welfare, and the third on schools as a service delivery sector to promote children's mental health.

NIMH currently has two standing program announcements (PAs) relevant to the dissemination and implementation of EBPs in child and adolescent mental health. The first, PA-02-131, entitled "Dissemination and Implementation Research in Mental Health," calls for "research that will build knowledge on methods, structures, and processes to disseminate and implement mental health information and treatments into practice settings." Research on dissemination is described to address how information about mental health care interventions is created, packaged, transmitted, and interpreted among various important stakeholder groups. Research on implementation is described to include a focus on the level to which mental health interventions can fit within real world mental health service systems. As of February 2004, there were 18 grants currently funded through this research program, including studies aimed at changing individual provider behavior, efforts to use technology to improve treatment and recovery for consumers with serious mental illness, and the use of consumer information on inpatient services to influence quality of care. A second PA, PA-04-019, "Practice, Effectiveness, and Implementation Research within the Center for Mental Health Services' (CMHS) Children's Service Sites," calls for research to be conducted within current or past CMHS-funded system of care or safe schools/healthy students grant communities. The announcement specifically encourages research on the implementation of evidence-based interventions for children within these grant communities.

A joint initiative (request for applications-MH-03-007) between NIMH and CMHS was launched in 2003 to support state mental health agency planning for research and service delivery agendas. Because each state has unique challenges, proposals that responded to the grant announcement were required to originate in a state agency, explain the challenges that the planning grant would tackle, and detail how specific planning activities would best enable the state to move forward. NIMH and CMHS equally contributed $1 million to fund nine 1-year planning grants. Of 38 peer-reviewed applications, state agencies from Arkansas, Maine, Maryland, Michigan, New York, North Carolina, Ohio, Texas, and Washington were awarded the planning grants. Topics of the grants ranged from general implementation of EBPS to age group–focused activities (eg, child, adult) to developing activities toward a specific diagnosis (eg, schizophrenia, depression). This is just the first step in establishing a robust body of knowledge about state-level implementation of EBPS, and each planning grant is expected to assist development of future NIMH and CMHS grant applications submitted by state agencies.

The Services Research and Clinical Epidemiology Branch at NIMH holds a bi-annual conference that spotlights advancement of the services research field regarding a specific theme. In 2002, this conference focused on the usefulness of evidence-based interventions in a theme entitled "Evidence in Mental Health Services Research: What Types, How Much, and Then What"? Last year, NIMH joined forces with the National Institute on Drug Abuse and the National Institute on Alcohol Abuse and Alcoholism on a conference that focused on the non-specialty mental health care sector, "Beyond the Clinic Walls: Expanding Mental Health, Drug and Alcohol Services Research Outside the Specialty Care System." This year's conference was entitled "Complexities of Co-occurring Conditions: Harnessing Services Research to Improve Care for Mental Illness, Substance Use, and Medical/Physical Disorders."

Center for Mental Health Services and Substance Abuse and Mental Health Services Administration

CMHS within the Substance Abuse and Mental Health Services Administration helps states improve and increase the quality and range of their treatment, rehabilitation, and support services for people with mental illness, their families, and communities. Substance Abuse and Mental Health Services Administration currently advocates the implementation of EBPs within funded communities (eg, safe schools/healthy students, systems of care).

CMHS currently provides funding to 61 communities under their comprehensive community mental health services program for children and families. This program is intended to encourage the development of home and community-based systems of care for children with serious emotional disturbances and their families. As a part of the national evaluation for the comprehensive community initiative, six randomized, controlled studies currently are being conducted. These trials are intended to evaluate evidence-based clinical interventions within several system of care sites. Two studies are devoted to each of the following interventions: parent-child interaction therapy, common sense parenting, and a substance abuse prevention program that targets seriously emotionally disturbed children. The overarching aim of these studies is to evaluate the degree to which such evidence-based intervention approaches enhance or detract from system of care outcomes for children served within these CMHS-funded communities.

CMHS also supports prevention service efforts across the country. As one example, the Targeted Capacity Expansion grant program strives to develop mental health prevention and early intervention services within community settings. Program goals include (1) expanding the capacity to implement evidence-based prevention programs and services, (2) building linkages with service providers, and (3) undertaking community outreach around community-based prevention. Grantees are asked to establish ongoing technical assistance relationships with evidence-based program developers and researchers and include intervention fidelity assessments within their implementation support system. Twenty-three grantees have received funding ($8.9 million) as of September, 2003.

CMHS also funds a $30 million initiative, the National Child Traumatic Stress Network. This network consists of a national coordinating center and 53 centers that collaboratively develop, implement, evaluate, and disseminate clinical treatments and trauma-informed service interventions for children and adolescents who experience traumatic events. The network is developing effective interventions for different types of trauma (eg, child maltreatment and domestic violence), different populations of traumatized children and adolescents (eg, preschool children, adolescents, rural youth), and use in community settings and in different child-serving service systems (eg, child mental health, child welfare, juvenile justice systems). The network operates through a set of committees organized under five core groupings—data, service systems, clinical interventions, training, and policy—to work on the improvement of traumatic stress service delivery.

Substance Abuse and Mental Health Services Administration also has maintained a national registry of effective practices and programs. The National Registry of Effective Practices and Programs began within the Center for Substance Abuse Prevention, and it focused on prevention programs with strong evidence of beneficial outcomes. Many of the programs that target children and adolescents (eg, multisystemic therapy, the Incredible Years program) also focus on the positive mental health of their client populations because of the strong correlation of risk factors between mental disorders and substance abuse. The National Registry of Effective Practices and Programs is being expanded beyond the Center for Substance Abuse Prevention to include mental health programs around three specific areas—mental health treatments for adults, mental health promotion and behavioral disorders prevention, and co-occurring (mental health and substance abuse) disorders.

Office of Special Education Programs, Office of Special Education and Rehabilitative Services, and Department of Education

The Office of Special Education Programs, Department of Education, housed in the Office of Special Education and Rehabilitative Services within the US Department of Education, works to improve results for infants, toddlers, children, and youth with disabilities by providing leadership and financial support to assist states and local districts. The Office of Special Education Programs has funded several centers of excellence that focus on children's mental health. These centers conduct research, provide technical assistance, develop training, and serve as networks to bridge the research and practice communities. Several centers primarily examine the social and emotional development of children. For instance, the Research and Training Center on Early Childhood Development at Orleana Hawks Puckett Institute in Asheville, North Carolina, seeks to translate the knowledge base on young children's early relationships, emotional, self-regulation, social development, and environmental factors into effective strategies that establish a foundation for school success. The research and training center also conducts effectiveness research, disseminates information on effective intervention practices, strategies, and methods, and provides training. The Office of Special Education Programs also funds two research centers for EBPs. The first, Project REACH at Lehigh University, focuses on children with intensive emotional, social, and behavioral needs. The other, the Center for Evidence-Based Practice at University of South Florida, focuses on young children with challenging behavior. Each center seeks to identify best and promising practices and conduct research to improve such services. The Office of Special Education Programs also sponsors a technical assistance center on positive behavioral intervention and supports. The center, administered by the University of Oregon in Eugene, focuses on capacity building and technical assistance to identify, adapt, and sustain effective school-wide disciplinary practices and provide broad dissemination to schools, families, and communities.

Office of Adolescent Health, Maternal and Child Health Bureau, and Health Resources and Services Administration

The Office of Adolescent Health, Maternal and Child Health Bureau within the Health Resources and Services Administration funds programs that aim to promote the health, development, safety, and social and emotional well-being of all school-aged children, adolescents, and young adults and their families. This office supports grants for national centers on school-based health care to provide current, evidence-based information and other resources to school-based and school-linked health centers. Two centers that focus on mental health in schools are currently being supported—one is at University of California, Los Angeles and the other is at University of Maryland, Baltimore. These centers provide technical assistance and training to persons interested in mental health in the schools and pursue a wide range of activities designed to improve how schools address barriers to learning and enhance healthy development. The center at University of California, Los Angeles focuses on the institutionalization and infrastructure support necessary to implement evidence-based practices. Some of the work at University of Maryland, Baltimore surrounding EBPs includes a review of the literature, identification of empirically supported interventions, and development of a resource packet to support EBPs in schools.

Child Outcomes Research and Evaluation, Office of Planning, Research and Evaluation, and Administration for Children and Families

The Administration for Children and Families is responsible for federal programs that promote the economic and social well-being of families, children, individuals, and communities. The Administration for Children and Families' Child Outcomes Research and Evaluation team within the Office of Planning, Research, and Evaluation provides scientific consultation, coordination, executive direction, and support for the implementation of short- and long-term research agendas within the administration. The Administration for Children and

Families funds Head Start and Early Head Start programs, which are comprehensive child development programs that serve children from birth to age 5, pregnant women, and their families.

In spring 1997, the Administration for Children and Families began the Family and Child Experiences Survey, a national longitudinal study of the cognitive, social, emotional, and physical development of Head Start children; the characteristics, well-being, and accomplishments of families; the observed quality of Head Start classrooms; and the characteristics, needs, and opinions of Head Start teachers and other program staff. Data collection took place annually each spring for the initial sample, including follow-up for kindergarten and first-grade children who completed Head Start. In fall 2000, a new cohort of Family and Child Experiences Survey was launched, with 2800 children in 43 new Head Start programs. Although the assessments of children were comprehensive, reaching beyond mental health outcomes, the study team did use evidence-based measures where available.

The Head Start mental health consortium, which began in the late 1990s, targeted five linked programs to promote evidence-based assessments and services for young children. The Walker Early Screening Program was adapted for use with various minority populations, and several rigorously examined programs that targeted children with disruptive behavior problems and children with language and behavior problems were delivered and assessed within a range of Head Start settings. A common dataset that measures levels of mental health and educational functioning across the five programs has been created and is being examined.

Office of Juvenile Justice and Delinquency Prevention, Office of Justice Programs, and United States Department of Justice

The Office of Juvenile Justice and Delinquency Prevention (OJJDP) supports states and communities in their efforts to develop and implement effective and coordinated prevention and intervention programs and improve the juvenile justice system. In August 2001, OJJDP invested $1 million in a new initiative to create a model for the delivery of mental health and related substance abuse services to youth within the juvenile justice system. The project received additional funding of $500,000 by OJJDP and the Substance Abuse and Mental Health Services Administration in 2003. Researchers from Policy Research Associates, Inc. conducted a literature review of theory and best practices for screening, assessment, service provision, and quality assurance, conducted a survey of mental health needs and services among youth in selected regions, and site visited promising programs around the country. Based on these activities, a service delivery model currently is being developed to encompass all stages related to the processing of youth in the juvenile justice system, including initial police contact and arrest, intake, detention, adjudication, disposition, placement, probation, and aftercare services.

OJJDP also offered support to an ongoing project based at the Center for the Study and Prevention of Violence at the University of Colorado, Boulder that identified model programs for violence prevention and worked to connect interested communities with program developers to help sites choose and implement a set of programs as effectively as possible. This initiative, entitled the "Blueprints Project," evolved into a large-scale prevention initiative, with 11 model programs and an additional 21 promising programs. More than 600 programs have been reviewed, and technical assistance has been offered to program developers and community settings. The Center for the Study and Prevention of Violence continues to work toward building the body of knowledge on implementation by keeping track of each "Blueprints" program site. OJJDP's contribution has provided funding for training and technical assistance for replications of the "Blueprints" programs at more than 42 sites around the United States.

Foundation efforts

Many of the private foundations have initiatives that focus on the improvement of mental health for children and adolescents. Each foundation has taken its own strategy, whether through funding research, document creation, or service demonstration projects, and significant progress has been made. We provide a brief summary of some of the work in which foundations are engaged currently.

John D. and Catherine T. MacArthur Foundation

The gap between science and practice has been widely acknowledged and documented. Treatments that have been shown to be effective in ameliorating mental health problems through clinical trials tend to be applied only in additional clinical trials, not in clinical practice. The John D. and Catherine T. MacArthur Foundation aims to reduce inequities in access to mental health services and bridge the gap between policy and practice. The MacArthur foundation supports several child mental health activities, but their primary initiative in children's mental health supports a network of child mental health experts. This group represents the fields of psychology, pediatrics, psychiatry, sociology, social work, and statistics to examine the gap between psychosocial intervention research findings and ongoing community-based mental health services for children. This includes an examination of inadequate financing, inappropriately designed benefits, and fragmentation of services.

The network has instituted a 4-year study that consists of two complementary, parallel multisite research projects. A clinic treatment project will test two alternative methods of delivering EBPs within public community-based mental health clinics using training and supervision procedures designed for the settings and users. The researchers are testing two different approaches to organizing and delivering EBPs: standard manuals, used exactly as they were originally tested in clinical trials, and modular manuals that can be individualized for each child using a guiding clinical algorithm. The clinic systems project will investigate the organizational, system, and payment issues that influence the ability of providers and clinics to use EBPs. The findings of these two projects will be used to plan a later phase of the work: disseminating EBPS to a broad array of clinics, providers, youths, and families and assessing the impact.

Klingenstein, Lowenstein, and Kellogg Foundations

The Klingenstein Third Generation Foundation has initiated a series of projects to improve the quality of school mental health services. For example, on December 3–4, 2003, the Klingenstein Foundation, along with co-sponsors Lowenstein Foundation and Kellogg Foundation, sponsored a 2-day national conference to highlight key issues involved in disseminating and implementing EBPs in school settings. This conference included national research and policy experts on school mental health, key advocacy organizations, and state and local leaders in school reform. The purpose of the conference was to examine strategies for promoting and strengthening school mental health across national, state, and local levels. A set of strategic opportunities was identified, and a coalition of professional mental health associations, advocacy organizations, and research scientists on school mental health are currently undertaking a series of multisite research and coalition-building activities to strengthen and support local, state, and national efforts to bridge education and mental health.

Annie E. Casey Foundation

Foundation initiatives also focus on disseminating EBPs by melding training and supervisory models across different sets of interventions. The Annie E. Casey Foundation's primary mission is to foster public policies, human service reforms, and community supports that more effectively meet the needs of vulnerable children and families. The foundation, through its BlueSky Project, has engaged the developers of three high-intensity interventions for youth with disruptive behavior problems (multisystemic therapy, multidimensional treatment foster care, and functional family therapy) to create a continuum of care that involves provisions of the preceding interventions for such youth. This program has received funding to focus on the implementation of these interventions designed for disadvantaged youth in the juvenile justice system. The foundation is developing a prototype model for implementation in two to three states by September 2004. The Annie E. Casey Foundation anticipates future funds for model implementation and will require that states meet several requirements to implement the prototype: current implementation of one of the interventions flexibility in funding (reallocation of funds for the project), and supportive placement decisions or referrals from judges and others in the system.

Annenberg Foundation Trust at Sunnylands

The Annenberg Foundation Trust at Sunnylands exists to advance the well-being of democratic institutions and enhance civic engagement and mental health

among youth. In 2001, the Annenberg Foundation Trust at Sunnylands established the adolescent mental health initiative, a joint venture with the Annenberg
Public Policy Center of the University of Pennsylvania. The initiative, which has
$6 million of committed funds from the foundation, set up six commissions to
compile and evaluate available research on several adolescent mental health
disorders—anxiety, schizophrenia, substance and alcohol abuse, depression and
bipolar disorder, eating disorders, and suicide—and an additional commission to
focus on positive youth development to underscore the prevention of these disorders in adolescence.

Each commission is responsible for the creation of a consensus document that
addresses the content of the disorder (clinical presentation, phenomenology,
neurobiology, genetics, pathophysiology) and guidelines for treatment and
prevention. The documents will compile the most current information about
each disorder and identify gaps in the research to set future research agendas for
the field in each area. A comprehensive book with the findings of all the com-
missions, written for mental health practitioners and researchers, is scheduled to
come out in early 2005. Books for other audiences (eg, teachers, parents, school
counselors) are also under development.

Commonwealth Fund

The Commonwealth Fund supports independent research on health issues and
makes grants to improve health care access and quality. One aspect of the
Commonwealth Fund's work centers on promoting young children's social and
emotional development and reducing the rate of childhood mental health disorders. Although the foundation supports EBPs, their focus on preventive
pediatric care (a poorly researched area) necessitates promoting the creation of
new models that use scientifically based practices. For instance, the assuring
better child development initiative supports state Medicaid programs to improve
delivery and financing of services (eg, screening and assessment, anticipatory
education, referral and care coordination) to promote better child development.
Four states (North Carolina, Vermont, Utah, and Washington) were funded in
Phase One for three years, receiving $100,000 each year. Phase Two is underway,
with five states (California, Illinois, Iowa, Minnesota, and Utah) receiving
funding ($55,000 per year for 3 years) to create models to enhance healthy
mental development for children, aged 0 to 3, and develop programs and policies
that ensure that health plans and providers who serve these children have the
skills to foster healthy development effectively.

State initiatives

Although a formal survey of evidence-based initiatives has not been conducted and soon would be out of date, we present a brief summary of some state
initiatives currently underway. These initiatives, all unique in their own ways, are

designed to create state-level strategies for disseminating a single or several EBPs or engage in comprehensive training, supervisory, or regulatory activities to implement a range of EBPs across the broad range of childhood disorders.

New York

New York is implementing a range of EBPs across the state and is engaged in a major effort to evaluate the impact of the implementation processes. For example, functional family therapy, a research-based treatment for youth with antisocial behavior problems and delinquency, is being implemented in approximately 12 sites statewide, after an active process of community involvement that sought stakeholder input about needs and options. Another large-scale implementation effort is being undertaken in New York to implement and evaluate a set of evidence-based trauma treatments for 350 youth affected by the World Trade Center disaster on September 11, 2001. New York State also has created a research bureau that focuses specifically on EBPs for children and adolescents to track the implementation of research-based services broadly defined, to include research-based assessment tools, engagement strategies [6], and a range of specific scientifically supported treatment models and assessment practices in school and mental health clinics. New York also has been awarded one of the NIMH Substance Abuse and Mental Health Services Administration state planning grants to develop a set of tools and methodologic approaches for assessing the fit between specific EBP models and organizational and contextual factors within mental health clinics and schools statewide. The focus of this effort is to improve understanding of family and consumer perspectives on organizational issues relevant to the adoption of new clinical practices.

Texas

A different strategy has been undertaken in Texas, which is seeking to formulate a benefit package of selected EBPs to be supported through training and monitoring. A consensus conference made up of family advocates, policy makers, clinical practitioners, and treatment and service model developers assisted the state in designing a new benefit package for youth that would include diagnostic-specific psychotherapies and comprehensive community-based services to address the full range of mental health needs of youth and families. This benefit design was implemented in 2003.

Michigan

In Michigan, a state planning process led to the identification of two interventions to address the most common clinical problems, with a plan to train practitioners to provide cognitive behavior therapy for internalizing disorders (with assistance from University of California, Los Angeles) and parent management training to address externalizing disorders (with assistance from the Oregon Social Learning Center).

Kentucky

CMHS, in conjunction with its children's services grant program, is adding EBPs to systems of care established under this program. Formal implementation of an EBPS is occurring in eastern Kentucky, where parent-child interaction treatment has been added to a system of care site. Although many randomized clinical trials of parent-child interaction treatment have been conducted, this is the first time that one will be conducted outside of academia. Parent-child interaction treatment is being randomized to schools and will be implemented in a large county in Oregon, where mental health centers will be the locus of treatment.

Ohio and California

CMHS also is funding EBP implementation initiatives in Ohio and California, which have been working on achieving buy-in from multiple stakeholder groups in each county. Ohio, through its Center on Innovative Practices, is implementing multisystemic therapy, intensive home-based services, and wraparound services. California, through the California Institute of Mental Health, is implementing treatment foster care, functional family therapy, and Webster-Stratton's Incredible Years through involvement with multiple service sectors.

Hawaii

An ambitious dissemination approach has been undertaken in Hawaii, called the Hawaii Experiment. The combination of a 14-month review of the research literature on psychosocial treatments for youth by a group of stakeholders, including families, policy makers, researchers, and practitioners, identified a set of treatments that have been systematically deployed in Hawaiian schools. A partnership between academia and the state led to the implementation of EBPs and a process of distillation of a set of EBPs into core practice components [7]. This process of distillation has enabled more clinician flexibility in selecting components of treatments that fit with parent, child, and clinical needs. This statewide initiative is being monitored carefully with respect to treatment planning, service provision, and outcomes.

Discussion

Next steps

Although much progress has been made toward building an evidence base around the effective dissemination and implementation of EBPs for children who experience emotional disorders, we have tremendous opportunities to move the field further. We are excited to see federal, state, and foundation initiatives not only to establish the efficacy of interventions but also to help build our knowledge about the actual processes involved in bringing these interventions into appropriate real world use. This new era of science and service likely will bring with it unique challenges. We would like to discuss briefly some considerations for future efforts.

Better scientific understanding of dissemination and implementation processes

Interest in implementing EBPs is growing on local, state, and national levels, but efforts are currently constrained by limited resources and a lack of knowledge regarding how to integrate EBPs within complex, dynamic service systems. Large challenges also remain in "scaling up" interventions from a collection of individual sites to statewide and nationwide implementation. Because many agency initiatives remain committed to bringing scientifically supported interventions into practice, our scientific understanding of how best to do this at every level of our service delivery systems remains unacceptably weak.

Increased clarity around definitions and terms

Definitions of EBPs and criteria to meet this standard vary across scientific reviews [8] and EBP lists. For instance, some EBP lists take implementation feasibility into account, whereas others do not. Agencies also differ in their perceived roles within the EBP movement. Many of the institutes at the National Institutes of Health maintain responsibility for providing research to build an intervention science knowledge base but not for classifying interventions into EBP categories. Other federal and foundation initiatives have created categories, commissioned reviews of current evidence, and promoted the implementation of acceptable evidence-based interventions. Sometimes, selected interventions are dictated by the organization in the announcement of an initiative; other times, intervention selection criteria are described. The impact of an intervention being included on an EBP list is demonstrable; inclusion affords the intervention increased recognition and wider dissemination possibilities. Clearly it is important to communicate information about efficacious interventions to practice communities; however, we see a need to clarify selection standards better and communicate the strengths and limitations of EBP learned through our emerging implementation knowledge base.

Clarifying processes of dissemination, implementation, and diffusion

Given the frequency with which the processes of diffusion, dissemination, and implementation are used and the confusion among the terms to represent efforts to bring EBPs into local settings, more clarity is needed to distinguish each process. Although more dialog is needed to reach consensus on the boundaries and specifics of each term, working definitions have been set through the NIMH program announcement "Dissemination and Implementation Research in Mental Health" [9] to start discussion toward eventual consensus:

Within this announcement, dissemination is defined as the targeted distribution of a well-defined set of information (eg, information about a health treatment). As Bauchner and Simpson [10] stated, "Dissemination is the active process of making information available to the target audience. It is the process

by which knowledge is made accessible or available to a particular audience."
The success of a dissemination effort can be measured by assessing whether the
audience received the information and whether the information was consistent
throughout the dissemination process.

By contrast, implementation is defined as the process of introducing or
changing practice into a specific local setting [9]. Implementation focuses on
the specific effort to fit a program, treatment, device, or procedure within a specific care context. It is distinguished from dissemination by its focus on the
individual fit of a "practice" into a specific setting. Wide-scale implementation
across multiple sites is greatly needed by the field, and the use of the term "implementation" acknowledges the importance of understanding each context in which
the practice is introduced.

Diffusion is defined as the intended and unintended spread of information or
treatments throughout the health services field. This umbrella term encompasses
all ways in which information and practices are spread throughout the field,
including those as the result of a targeted effort and those communicated in-
directly (eg, informal chats, case conferences). This enables an understanding of
the degree to which information and practices are used throughout the field (often
referred to in management as "market penetration") and accounts for all ways in
which information and practices are transmitted. The distinctions among dissemination, implementation, and diffusion are made to acknowledge the different
degrees of effort required to bring science into practice.

Increased efforts to build infrastructure and support policy change

Most federal, foundation, and state efforts have focused on the implementation
of specific clinical-level interventions. These efforts have led to an increased
understanding of the difficulties associated with implementing an evidence-based
program into a complex, resource-limited care setting. Given the demands on
staff, limited resources, and instability of mental health care organizations, even
more challenging is the sustainability of the program over time. Factors that
often impact program change or intervention sustainability have to do with an
overarching infrastructure (eg, reimbursement policies, staff training, administrative support). There is a need for increased efforts to review effective ways in
which communities (at the state or local level) have surmounted these infrastructure challenges. Such efforts ideally will facilitate our knowledge not only about
how to implement such practices but also how to keep them operating well for the
long-term.

Identification and use of nonclinical evidence-based practices to support
implementation

The EBP term seems to be associated most often with reviews of client-level
(child or family) interventions. Based on our brief review, this term is rarely
applied to system or organization-level interventions (eg, quality assurance

methods). Is it possible to include EBPs to refer to system-level interventions to improve and sustain client-level interventions? Our emerging knowledge about successful implementation efforts suggests that the environment within which an intervention is placed has an impact on eventual program outcomes. Meanwhile, we seldom include in our discussion of EBPs the systemic efforts that are necessary to support efficacious intervention approaches. New initiatives that incorporate knowledge about how to build an infrastructure to support high-quality mental health interventions are absolutely critical.

Expansion of client-level intervention studies to include systemic outcomes

In addition to the need to identify system-level interventions that support the implementation of EBPs, we need the client-level interventions to incorporate system-level outcomes as targets of the interventions. The need to fit a client-level intervention within a complex service system should be addressed better by intervention developers, because existing system interventions may not always fit with treatment program characteristics. A melding of client-level and system-level targets likely would improve the usefulness of evidence-based interventions.

Aggregation of anecdotal data on implementing evidence-based practices

In recent years, many initiatives have sought to implement EBPs into real world clinical settings. As this article has shown, on virtually every level of the mental health care system (national, state, and local) and in every sector (public and private), implementers have learned a great deal about the strengths and limitations of implementation strategies. The field would benefit greatly from some organized "farming" of this experiential data gleaned from all of these initiatives. Without some ability to share reflections across EBPs, clinical settings, and public and private organizations, little will be learned from these significant endeavors. A group of researchers in the United Kingdom has sought to aggregate data from case studies that examine evidence-based medicine [11]. A similar effort should be undertaken in mental health.

Summary

The breadth and number of federal, foundation, and state initiatives in this area is exciting. Given the President's New Freedom Commission report description of the US mental health system as "fragmented and in disarray" [3], it is vitally important that attempts be made to improve on the care provided to children with mental disorders and behavioral and emotional problems. The federal, foundation, and state initiatives described in this article are important steps in the right direction and should enable the improvement of services within the child and adolescent mental health system and the knowledge base from which to further improve mental health.

Acknowledgments

The authors wish to thank the following individuals for their assistance in the writing of the manuscript: Gary Blau, PhD, Center for Mental Health Services, Substance Abuse and Mental Health Services Administration; Renee Bradley, PhD, Office of Special Education Programs, Department of Education; Sybil Goldman, PhD, Center for Mental Health Services, Substance Abuse and Mental Health Services Administration; Malcolm Gordon, PhD, Center for Mental Health Services, Substance Abuse and Mental Health Services Administration; Isadora Hare, MSW, Health Resources and Services Administration; Tom Hanley, EdD, Office of Special Education Programs, Department of Education; Seth Hassett, MSW, Center for Mental Health Services, Substance Abuse and Mental Health Services Administration; Kelly Henderson, PhD, Office of Special Education Programs, Department of Education; Kathleen Hall Jamieson, PhD, Annenberg Trust at Sunnylands; Michael Lopez, PhD, Administration for Children and Families; Patrick McCarthy, PhD, Annie E. Casey Foundation; Constance M. Pechura, PhD, Robert Wood Johnson Foundation; Melissa Racioppo, PhD, National Institute on Drug Abuse; Edward L. Schor, MD, Commonwealth Fund; Rolando Santiago, PhD, Center for Mental Health Services, Substance Abuse and Mental Health Services Administration; Kyle Snow, PhD, National Institute of Child Health and Human Development; Karen Stern, PhD, Office of Juvenile Justice and Delinquency Prevention; Louisa B. Tarullo, EdD, Administration for Children and Families.

References

[1] Lonigan CJ, Elbert JC, Johnson SB. Empirically supported psychosocial interventions for children: an overview. J Clin Child Psychol 1998;27:138–45.

[2] Hoagwood K, Burns BJ, Kiser L, Ringeisen H, Schoenwald SK. Evidence-based practice in child and adolescent mental health services. Psychiatr Serv 2001;52(9):1179–89.

[3] President's New Freedom Commission on Mental Health. Achieving the promise: transforming mental health care in America: final report. Publication no. SMA-03–3832. Rockville: Department of Health and Human Services; 2003.

[4] US Public Health Service. Report of the surgeon general's conference on children's mental health: a national action agenda. Washington, DC: US Publica Health Service; 2000.

[5] National Advisory Mental Health Council's Workgroup on Child and Adolescent Mental Health Intervention and Deployment. Blueprint for change: research on child and adolescent mental health. Publication 01–4985. Rockville: National Institute of Mental Health; 2001.

[6] McKay M, Bannon W. Engaging families in child mental health services. Child Adolesc Psychiatric Clin North Am 2004;13(4):905–21.

[7] Chorpita BF, Yim LM, Donkervoet JC, Arensdorf A, Amundsen MJ, McGee C, et al. Toward large-scale implementation of empirically supported treatments for children: a review and observations by the Hawaii empirical basis to services task force. Clinical Psychology Science and Practice 2002;9(2):165–90.

[8] Drake R, Goldman H, Leff H, Lehman A, Dixon L, Mueser K, et al. Implementing evidence-based practices into routine mental health service settings. Psychiatr Serv 2001;52(2): 179–82.

[9] National Institute of Mental Health. Dissemination and implementation research in mental

health. Available at: http://grants.nih.gov/grants/guide/pa-files/PA-02-131.html. Accessed March 31, 2004.

[10] Bauchner H, Simpson L. Specific issues related to developing, disseminating, and implementing pediatric practice guidelines for physicians, patients, families, and other stakeholders. Health Serv Res 1998;33(4):1161–77.

[11] Ferlie E, Gabbay J, Fitzgerald L, Locock L, Dopson S. Evidence-based medicine and organisational change: an overview of some recent qualitative research. In: Ashburner L, editor. Organisational behaviour and organisational studies in health care: reflections on the future. London: Palgrave; 2001. p. 18–42.

ELSEVIER
SAUNDERS

Child Adolesc Psychiatric Clin N Am
14 (2005) 329–349

CHILD AND
ADOLESCENT
PSYCHIATRIC CLINICS
OF NORTH AMERICA

From Data to Wisdom: Quality Improvement Strategies Supporting Large-scale Implementation of Evidence-Based Services

Eric L. Daleiden, PhD[a,b,*], Bruce F. Chorpita, PhD[c]

[a]*Child and Adolescent Mental Health Division, Hawaii Department of Health, 3627 Kilauea Avenue, Room101, Honolulu, HI 96816, USA*
[b]*Department of Psychiatry, John A. Burns School of Medicine, University of Hawaii at Manoa, 2430 Campus Road, Honolulu, HI 96825, USA*
[c]*Department of Psychology, University of Hawaii at Manoa, 2430 Campus Road, Honolulu, HI 96825, USA*

The goal of this article is to illustrate various strategies that the Hawaii Child and Adolescent Mental Health Division (CAMHD) adopted to increase the use of empirical evidence to improve the quality of services and outcomes for youth. We operate from the premise that evidence-based decision making extends beyond the use of treatment outcome literature to inform decisions regarding treatment selection. We elaborate a list of common clinical decisions, discuss multiple evidence bases that may inform these decisions, and use a model of the phases of evidence to illustrate multiple quality improvement strategies used within the Hawaii system of care for youth. This article provides a broad overview to various quality initiatives for promoting evidence-based practices rather than in-depth discussion of any specific strategy.

Background

Major systems reform has pervaded the Hawaii system of care for youth for more than a decade. Two federal lawsuits played important roles in promoting

---

* Corresponding author. Child and Adolescent Mental Health Division, Hawaii Department of Health, 3627 Kilauea Avenue, Room101, Honolulu, HI 96816.
E-mail address: eldaleid@camhmis.health.state.hi.us (E.L. Daleiden).

childpsych.theclinics.com

these developments. First, in 1991, the State of Hawaii settled a class action lawsuit with the US Department of Justice for violations of the civil rights of individuals residing at Hawaii State Hospital. Second, in 1994, because of a failure to provide necessary mental health and educational services as required by the Individuals with Disabilities in Education Act and Section 504 of the Rehabilitation Act, the federal courts enjoined the State of Hawaii Departments of Health and Education in the Felix Consent Decree. The state was charged with establishing a system of care to provide effective mental health and special education services for children and youth in need of such services to benefit from their education.

Following a large-scale community planning effort, the early system response to these directives focused on building service capacity, promoting multi-agency coordination, and establishing quality monitoring. Implementation of these reforms yielded large increases in the number of youth accessing services, the amount and type of services available, and the total expenditures for mental health services. The statewide quality monitoring structure relied heavily on system and child reviews performed by interagency monitoring teams [1] and developing information systems to manage child registrations, service authorizations, electronic billing, and claims adjudication. The output of this quality system was extensive qualitative and rudimentary quantitative feedback to stakeholders during review debriefing sessions and management reports illustrating the increasing population, services, and expenses.

With these successes in place, the reform focus evolved to questioning if the expanded investment contributed to improved outcomes. Large-scale dissemination of evidence-based services was explored as an initiative to improve child outcomes [2]. Stakeholders also wanted assurances of resource efficiency and services that effectively improved lives. Empirical evidence again was sought as the arbiter of claims. To support continued system development, the focus of the Hawaii CAMHD shifted to identifying (1) clinical decisions that could be more evidence based, (2) evidence bases that could support these decisions, and (3) approaches for linking the evidence bases to the decision making. CAMHD efforts have targeted administrative and clinical processes, but this article focuses on evidence-based clinical decision making. This discussion may be readily generalized to the business context.

Core clinical decisions

Many decisions are made on a daily basis in the clinical context. A fundamental strategic concern for system management is clarifying priorities regarding which common decisions should be targeted for systemic development. Some common clinical decisions include (1) where to treat clients, (2) how to treat clients, (3) who should treat clients, (4) whether quality services are being provided to clients, (5) whether clients are getting better, (6) how to manage and supervise treatment, (7) who should make the decisions. These decisions by no means constitute a comprehensive list but represent many of the perennial questions faced by CAMHD.

When designing a comprehensive treatment system that serves diverse consumer populations across many settings and through numerous service agencies and service providers, one is faced with the strategic decision of whether to build evidence bases to educate individual decisions or to package these decisions in some meaningful fashion. The empirically supported treatment movement has headed strongly in the direction of packaging decisions into structured treatment programs, so that the single choice about which treatment program to select guides the answer to the other core questions. For example, the evidence-based multisystemic therapy program is designed to serve youth in the home and community setting using family therapy and behavioral techniques, measure quality using therapist and supervisor adherence measures, monitor instrumental and ultimate outcomes, and provide these services through treatment teams, team supervisors, and a higher level cross-team supervisor [3]. The fundamental choice to use the multisystemic therapy program essentially answers the other questions about where to treat, how to treat, who should treat, how to determine quality and outcomes, and how to manage the services.

As a brief aside, the decision-making circumstance at the individual clinician level generally differs from the systemic and programmatic decision-making situations. For example, a systemic treatment selection decision may be "Given the characteristics of the client population seeking services, the outcomes the system is trying to achieve, the available funding, the available workforce (eg, agencies and providers), and the capacity for workforce/provider development, what treatment programs should be made available to clinicians and consumers?" The resulting system design may function to constrain the options from which an individual clinician can choose. For example, if a system is designed so that clinicians operate within settings (eg, outpatient versus residential) but across populations and programs, a clinician's key treatment selection question may be "Given my context (eg, outpatient setting), my client's characteristics (eg, 17-year-old girl), and the target for my consumer's treatment (eg, depressed and withdrawn behavior), what treatment program should be selected (eg, medication, interpersonal psychotherapy for adolescents [4], or adolescent coping with depression [5])?" It is beyond the scope of this article to address the multitude of forms the treatment selection decision may take, but the complexities associated with the diversity of decision contexts across analytic levels are important to keep in mind.

Returning to our main theme that the treatment selection decision fundamentally guides other core clinical decisions when a treatment system is designed at the program level, building an evidence base to educate the treatment selection decision may be viewed as a proxy for building many evidence bases needed to educate these other core decisions. Once the treatment program is selected, systemic quality management often focuses on whether the appropriate clientele are accessing the service, whether treatment programs are implemented with integrity to their design (ie, whether the subsequent core decisions are being answered as programmatically specified), and whether sufficient resources (eg, workforce, skills, funding) exist to support the system. Program-based design may become problematic at the system level if each program uses different quality measures, different outcome measures, and different management structures. At the individual provider/consumer level, program-based design may become problematic when youth characteristics are a poor match with program focus and when youth have completed all the best programs but remain in need of service. Based on this type of analysis, CAMHD staff reasoned that the treatment selection decision was a good place to start building evidence-based clinical decision making but that the system also needed to move beyond the selection decision to inform the additional decisions systematically.

In CAMHD's analysis, three common models for treatment selection were identified, namely the evidence-based services model, the individualized case conceptualization model, and the practice-based evidence model. These models rely on four common evidence bases to inform the treatment selection decision. The evidence-based services model relies on evidence from the general services and intervention research literatures to identify treatments with scientific support for their efficacy and effectiveness. The individualized case conceptualization model relies on case-specific historical evidence and evidence of the general causal mechanisms underlying the problem at hand. The practice-based evidence model relies on case-specific historical evidence that is locally aggregated to identify relevant treatments that have worked best with similar cases in the local system. Although these models are oversimplified in this article, they highlight the four key evidence bases that may inform treatment selection.

CAMHD views each of these evidence bases as providing important information, but each also has notable limitations. Currently, any single model is insufficient for system management because of gaps in the available evidence and biases in clinical decision making [6]. These different models require integration into a full system model (Fig. 1) to best inform the multitude of decisions by the different stakeholders that are a routine part of clinical service delivery. Fig. 1 conceptually illustrates that four key databases are used to assist treatment teams (or individual providers, depending on system design) in making the core clinical decisions. To date, CAMHD's efforts have focused heavily on building strategies for three evidence bases (ie, case-specific history, local aggregate summaries, and general services and intervention research databases). We believe, however, that realizing the long-term potential for mental health services lies in the development and delivery of knowledge from the fourth evidence base about the causal mechanisms underlying psychopathology and recovery.

A common issue across the three treatment selection models (ie, evidence-based services, individualized case conceptualization, and practice-based evidence models) is that of the appropriate basis for matching interventions to individual youth. In one of its most salient forms, this often presents as the question of whether diagnosis should serve as the basis for treatment selection. Addressing the nuances of this issue is beyond the scope of this article, and differing perspectives continue to be represented within the CAMHD system [7].

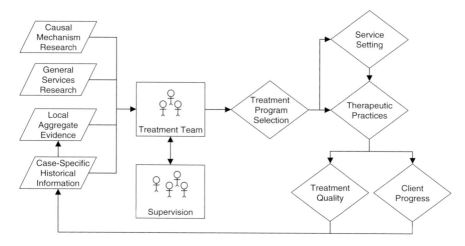

Fig. 1. System model that illustrates the four core evidence bases and their relation to key service decisions.

The CAMHD analysis has tended to focus on treatment targets, not just diagnosis, as a core driver of treatment selection. Relevant treatment targets are identified during service planning, are negotiated with consumers and professionals, and are related to, but distinct from, diagnoses. This is not a traditional model in which diagnosis is the focus of treatment and the service goal is elimination of the disorder that causes impairment. Instead, diagnosis is viewed as a key proxy variable that summarizes common targets for change, highlights plausible etiologic pathways, and serves as an important contextual factor for matching interventions to targets.

For example, a preadolescent boy with a diagnosis of attention deficit hyperactivity disorder and his family may seek home-based services to improve academic achievement and increase positive family functioning. In this case, the set of relevant treatments include those found to improve academic and family functioning in contexts that approximate the characteristics of the current case (ie, preadolescent boy diagnosed with attention deficit hyperactivity disorder, home-based setting). On the other hand, treatments that reduce symptoms of attention deficit hyperactivity disorder (eg, attention, hyperactivity) but do not alter academic or family functioning might not be considered despite the fact that the treatment matches the case on primary diagnosis.

At the system design level, this example highlights the importance of understanding the common targets of interest to relevant stakeholders when selecting interventions. For example, because of its relationship with the department of education, academic achievement might be a much more common target of intervention for the CAMHD population than is typical in other service systems. Accordingly, designing the system to include programs that improve academic functioning is a high priority.

Managing evidence bases

When designing and managing evidence bases to support clinical decision making, CAMHD staff have found two general frameworks to be useful. First, CAMHD attempts to apply basic scientific values and evaluate proposed developments against the criteria of whether they will be structured, reliable, valid, useful, publicly verifiable, distributable, and self-correcting over the long run [8].

A second useful framework describes the phases of evidence as data, information, knowledge, and wisdom [9]. Data refer to discretely identifiable units; information is data represented in a context that provides meaning; knowledge is information that is helpful for decision making; and wisdom is awareness of when to apply knowledge. When applied to developing evidence bases, this model highlights the activities of defining and capturing relevant data, organizing and analyzing it into meaningful units for consumers, delivering the information to the decision-making situation, and prioritizing use of the knowledge bases. In analogy, the quality improvement system acts as a video camera (focusing on each of the evidence bases) and as a video monitor (delivering the relevant information at the locus of decision making).

The remainder of this article focuses on illustrating the strategies that CAMHD uses to manage evidence-based clinical decision making. The phases of evidence framework is applied to the four relevant evidence bases identified previously. Finally, CAMHD's evidence-based clinical decision-making process is presented and illustrated.

Services research strategies

Hawaii's system of care for youth maintains an interagency evidence-based services committee that is responsible for reviewing the services research literature and providing guidance to decision makers [2,10]. This committee has identified at least two sources of relevant data: research articles and treatment protocols. The data from these sources are organized into information through the use of efficacy, effectiveness, and practice element codes. (For more details, the reader is referred elsewhere [2,7].) The methodology and results of research studies are used to assign treatments to a level system that describes the reliability of each treatment's efficacy. Various contextual features of the intervention (eg, setting, format, cost) are coded to aid in matching treatments to the decision makers' particular circumstance. Finally, the specific practices used within each protocol are coded to provide additional detail as to the protocol's procedural content and to promote practice profiling across studies.

Various strategies have been developed to deliver this information to the many decision-making contexts. One of the most widely adopted strategies has become affectionately known as the "blue menu." This one-page matrix summarizes evidence-based services with target problems in the rows, the efficacy level in the columns, and the description of the treatment packages in the cells (Table 1). Psychosocial treatments are represented on one side and psychopharmacologic interventions are on the other. Whereas the blue menu provides a roadmap to the efficacy level of various services, the biennial report of the evidence-based services committee provides detailed information on the full coding of the interventions and includes convenient reference tables, including information relevant to treatment contexts [10].

In addition to these direct summaries, service research information is incorporated into interagency performance standards and practice guidelines that serve as a contractual attachment when the system procures services for youth. These standards and guidelines are incorporated into ongoing performance and contract monitoring activities. CAMHD also maintains a practice development office that is responsible for providing interagency training, mentoring, and consultation to promote ongoing skill development and dissemination of service research information. Funding structures are also viewed as a mechanism for delivering service information to clinical decision makers. Although CAMHD has a flexible funding benefit that allows for construction of customized services when appropriate, many treatment teams initially elect to use the services included in the standing CAMHD service array. Developing long-term contracts with structured reimbursement protocols for evidence-based programs (eg, multisystemic therapy [3]) and including these programs in the routine service array increases the likelihood that they will be selected and be readily available as front-line treatments. Along with the performance monitoring activities mentioned previously, CAMHD has evolved its utilization management procedures to monitor whether relevant populations are receiving evidence-based levels of care and whether service usage is consistent with practice guidelines.

Case history strategies

CAMHD has targeted local case-specific data from regular clinical interactions in the form of clinical assessments, service authorizations, and billing records. A multitude of structures organize these data into information. Diagnoses from the "Diagnostic and Statistical Manual" [11] are used to summarize the complexities of clients' symptomatology and service plans organize treatment targets and interventions data. Quarterly standardized assessments are used to monitor symptomatology (Achenbach System of Empirically Based Assessment [12]), functioning (Child and Adolescent Functional Assessment Scale [13]), and service needs (Child and Adolescent Level of Care Utilization System [14]). Treatment providers complete a monthly summary that measures treatment settings, formats, targets, progress ratings, and practices using context and prac-

Table 1
Example of one-page summary of evidence-based child and adolescent psychosocial interventions. Hawaii's "Blue Menu"

Problem area	Level 1: Best support	Level 2: Good support	Level 3: Moderate support	Level 4: Minimal support	Level 5: Known risks
Anxious or avoidant behaviors	CBT: Exposure, modeling	CBT with parents, group cognitive behavior therapy, CBT for child and parent, educational support	None	Eye movement desensitization and reprocessing, play therapy, individual (supportive) therapy, group (supportive) therapy	None
Attention and hyperactivity behaviors	Behavior therapy	None	None	Biofeedback; play therapy, individual or group (supportive) therapy, social skills training, "Parents are Teacher," parent effectiveness training, self-control training	None
Autistic spectrum disorders	None	None	Applied behavior analysis, functional communication training, caregiver psychoeducation program	Auditory integration training, play therapy, individual or group (supportive) therapy	None
Bipolar disorder	None	Interpersonal and social rhythm therapy[a]	Family psychoeducational interventions[a]	All other psychosocial therapies	None
Depressive or withdrawn behaviors	CBT	CBT with parents, interpersonal therapy (manualized IPT-A), relaxation	None	Behavioral problem solving, family therapy, self-control training, self-modeling, and individual (supportive) therapy	None

Disruptive and oppositional behaviors	Parent and teacher training, PCIT	Anger coping therapy, assertiveness training, problem-solving skills training, rational emotive therapy, AC-SIT, PATHS, and FAST track programs	Social relations training, project achieve	Client-centered therapy, communication skills, goal setting, human relations therapy, relationship therapy, relaxation, stress inoculation, supportive attention	Group therapy
Eating disorders	CBT[a] (bulimia only)	Family therapy (anorexia only)	None	Individual (supportive) therapy	Some group therapy
Juvenile sex offenders	None	None	Multisystemic therapy[c]	Individual or group (supportive) therapy	Group therapy[c]
Delinquency and willful misconduct behavior	None	Multisystemic therapy	Multidimensional treatment foster care, wrap-around foster care	Individual therapy, juvenile justice system	Group therapy
Schizophrenia	None	None	Behavioral family management[a], family-based intervention[a], personal therapy[a], social interventions[a]	Supportive family management[a], applied family management[a]	None
Substance use	CBT[b]	Behavior therapy, purdue brief family therapy	None	Individual or group (supportive) therapy, interactional therapy, family drug education, conjoint family therapy, strategic structural systems engagement	Group therapy

This tool has been developed to guide teams (inclusive of youth, family, educators, and mental health practitioners) in developing appropriate plans using psychosocial interventions. Teams should use this information to prioritize promising options. For specific details about these interventions and their applications (eg, age setting, gender) see the most recent evidence-based services committee biennial report (http://www.hawaii.gov/health/mental-health/camhd/resources/index.html).

[a] Based on findings with adults only.

[b] Appropriate only if child is already in inpatient setting, otherwise consider level 2.

[c] If delinquency and willful misconduct are present.

tice element codes consistent with those used for the services research reviews by the evidence-based services committee.

A primary strategy for delivering this information to decision makers was the development of on-demand, user-friendly, graphics-based clinical reports in the management information system. Through an analogy with the instrument panel for driving a car, these reports have become known as the "clinical dashboards" for driving cases. To reduce demands on consumers and facilitate consistent communication, two figures were selected to represent all relevant data [15]. Adapted from single subject design representations [16], a line graph represents historical quantitative information, and a scatterplot represents historical qualitative information. Fig. 2 illustrates a global individual case summary that includes diagnosis, basic outcomes, interagency involvement, and the levels of care received. Users can "drill-down" into increasing depth of information, including scale scores, progress ratings, and even history of specific therapeutic practices. In addition to the on-line clinical reports, various operational reports also present case-specific information, such as sentinel event/critical incident reports, service gap and mismatch reports (eg, youth who have not received planned services within 30 days), and grievance reports.

As a cornerstone of its service monitoring activities, CAMHD uses case-based reviews [1] and administrative reviews. The annual review process uses small random samples from each region and each provider. A trained monitoring team reviews records, conducts interviews, and scores a structured case review protocol appropriate to the targeted service. Case-based reviews consume information from the standardized case reports described previously and generate unique information through use of a structured, multi-method review protocol and team-based review of the obtained data. In addition to written monitoring reports, debriefing sessions are conducted to deliver the knowledge to stakeholders, and action plans are developed when appropriate.

Incorporation of the standardized reports is encouraged (and in some instances required) at regular case presentations and practice reviews at the regional guidance centers, at clinical supervision, at individual service team meetings, and at various statewide professional development activities for the clinical leadership. Statewide practice development personnel and clinical leaders at the regional guidance centers also provide case-specific consultation and mentoring to front-line supervisors and service providers.

Local aggregate evidence strategies (practice-based evidence)

Local aggregate evidence is based on the same data sources as the case-specific evidence but is aggregated across cases into meaningful composite units. It is important to note, however, that administrative system transactions and operations also provide an important data source for aggregate evidence. For example, a timely credentialing transaction with a specific service provider may determine the availability of that provider for clinical intervention with a youth and may have implications for making decisions related to the youth's clinical

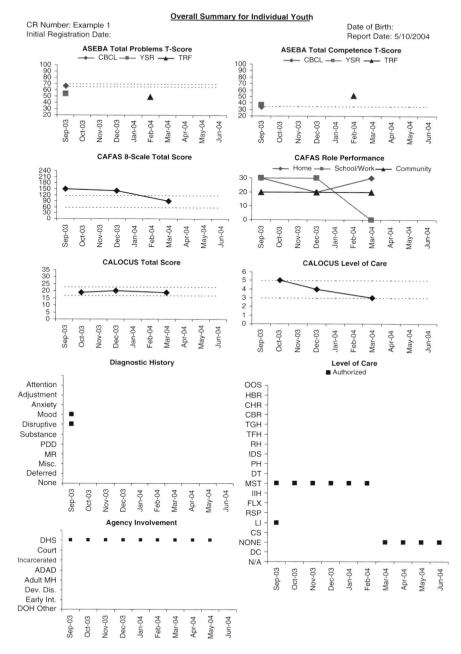

Fig. 2. Example of an overall case history report from the clinical report module of the Child and Adolescent Mental Health Management Information System.

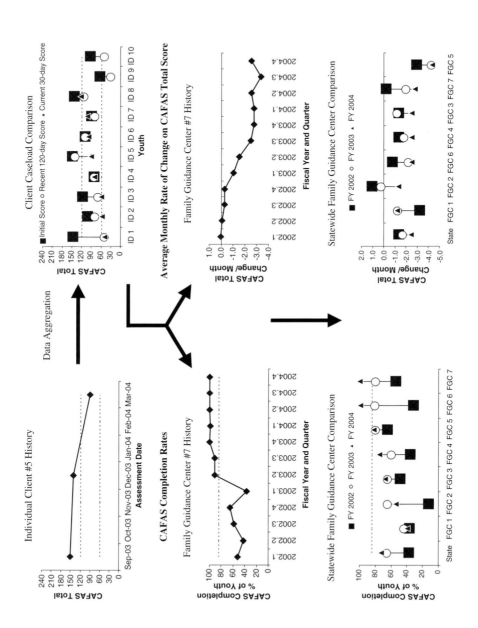

care. CAMHD tracks an extensive array of data on the quantity, timeliness, and quality of a diversity of administrative transactions, including the number of credentialing applications, the latency to credentialing process completion, and the number of errors in transactions between the credentialing office and the information system office.

Many of the strategies for organizing case history data into information also are used at the aggregate level (eg, diagnosis, standardized outcome measures). Aggregate data also are organized into information through the specification of performance measures [17]. A performance measure is a quantitative indicator of system functioning. Performance measures may be defined to assess the functioning of any component of a business process (eg, individual, group, business transaction, or clinical outcome). Most commonly, performance measures are indicators of the quantity, quality, timeliness, or consumer satisfaction with the targeted process. For example, data on number of applications and number of interoffice transaction errors may be organized into a monthly performance measure on the percent of credentialing transactions accepted on first submission by the information system office. This performance measure might be useful for educating personnel allocation, task training, and transaction format redesign decisions. Highly customized analysis and special studies of population, service, fiscal, performance, and outcome data are also used to organize aggregate data into information.

To deliver aggregated information, a standardized unit comparison dashboard was adopted. Fig. 3 illustrates the process of data aggregation through an alternation of the unit history and unit comparison dashboards. This illustration demonstrates how information on child functioning (lower scores indicate better functioning) is transformed and aggregated from an individual client history through a caseload report to two system performance measures on percent of youth with assessments completed during the quarter and the monthly average rate of change in functioning during the current treatment episode for youth served during the quarter. The unit comparison dashboard was designed to facilitate identification of common patterns across units and detection of atypical units for further review, whereas the unit history dashboard supports more in-depth review and detailed understanding. In the clinical reporting system, standardized clinical caseload reports are available on demand for quick analysis of cross-case patterns. Although not illustrated in this article, a standardized one-page presentation template that incorporates these dashboards is used for performance measure presentations. Performance measures are presented in verbal, visual, and written format on a regularly scheduled basis to designated managers and quality improvement committees.

Fig. 3. Example of how data are aggregated and displayed for the Child and Adolescent Functional Assessment Scale (CAFAS) from clinical client history and caseload reports to administrative performance measures for a regional family guidance center and for statewide comparison of performance trends across family guidance centers.

Several critiques of local aggregate evidence systems are common. First, data often are old and dated by the time they are collected, analyzed, and delivered in a usable format. Second, clinical and business problems may require short-term solutions that prohibit building and validating a new component of a large-scale information system. Third, if the speed of information delivery is accelerated, then the quality of information declines (ie, there is a speed-accuracy trade-off). Although CAMHD has made considerable progress in developing a timely and responsive statewide information system, much information remains to be integrated into the central information system. Special purpose information tools are produced in the form of stand-alone databases and spreadsheets designed to structure local data capture and provide immediate analysis and feedback using the standard dashboard presentation formats. Although regionally distributed, these tools are regularly collected and aggregated into statewide summaries. Although they do not support the integrity of the centralized information system, they provide a cost-effective, rapid development environment for information system innovations.

To deliver information from special studies, customized evaluation reports are written, summary slide shows are prepared, and results are presented to stakeholder groups, including designated quality improvement committees. When appropriate, findings are posted on the Internet for public reference. The quality improvement committees are responsible for making recommendations for action to executive management, who assign staff and resources to implement strategically selected actions. To facilitate interpersonal diffusion of information and develop diverse change agents [18], quality improvement committee members are recruited from broad stakeholder groups, including service consumers, providers, and personnel who represent assorted system functions. Regional branch chiefs also periodically extend broad invitations to stakeholders to attend public performance presentations. Finally, as with the services research, local aggregate evidence may inform best practice guidelines.

Causal mechanism strategies

The rapid expansion of the scientific literature and understanding of causes in the development of psychopathology offers considerable promise for improving the mental health of children. The past decades have witnessed increased coverage and availability of research studies through searchable computer database (eg, Educational Resources Information Center, Medline, PsychInfo) and increased access to expert knowledge through various telehealth programs. The President's New Freedom Commission on Mental Health [19] emphasized the importance of accelerating the progression from discovery to implementation of services in communities.

Currently, CAMHD relies heavily on its professional personnel to identify, consume, and apply knowledge of causal mechanisms. In addition to research articles, the training and experiences of the working professionals provide the core causal mechanism data. These data are organized into information through facts, theories, and opinions. The primary pathway for delivery of this information is the memory and judgment of treatment team members. This often is the most comprehensive evidence base that provides a rich breadth of knowledge where other evidence bases are lacking. For example, professional knowledge of causal mechanisms is often sought to construct interventions for treatment-resistant youth who have received the "best" empirically supported treatments but have not yet met treatment goals.

Despite this breadth of application, relying on individual professionals to gather and organize evidence related to causal mechanisms yields an evidence base that is unstandardized and variable in nature. As an evidence base, individual human memory and judgment fail to satisfy basic scientific values (eg, publicly verifiable), and information-processing biases may be the norm [6]. An opportunity seems to exist for improving the management of causal mechanism knowledge through improved information and communication systems that use structured protocols for monitoring, aggregating, and delivering causal evidence and facilitate its coordination within treatment teams (including youth and families). Managing the causal mechanism evidence base remains a relatively unexplored frontier for the CAMHD system.

Integrating the evidence: Hawaii's foray into wisdom

Fostering these evidence bases creates a data, information, and knowledge-rich environment. The next logical step is to build supports that allow decision makers to apply the "best" knowledge available to solve their current problem. This is wisdom, and it remains a precious resource. With the goal of wisdom clear in its sights, the CAMHD system has begun an initial venture into evidence-based clinical decision-making guidance. Among the many decision-making contexts, CAMHD has targeted clinical supervision as a primary application domain for integrating this broad array of evidence. Fig. 5 depicts a decision flow that is used to address several of the core clinical decisions.

When a new child enters the system, the first decision faced is that of treatment selection. The evidence-based decision-making flow prioritizes the services research evidence base and recommends use of the evidence-based service reports (ie, blue menu, biennial report) and practice guidelines to select an evidence-based service. For new cases, this choice most likely involves performing an assessment to generate case-specific evidence, followed by service planning that includes matching the newly acquired case evidence to a relevant evidence-based treatment. As services are implemented, ongoing supervision and case management address the question of whether significant concerns have emerged for the case. The decision guidance prioritizes review of case history evidence for critical incidents, such as sentinel events or grievances, and local aggregate evidence to determine the typical frequency of such incidents in the local environment. For example, if a few seclusion events are reported for the youth and local aggregate data indicate an elevated seclusion rate at a particular provider agency associated with temporarily increased staff vacancies, fundamental modification to treatment practices may be unnecessary in the short term. Alternatively, critical incidents without a contextual moderator may call for reconsideration of treatment selection or application of a specialists' causal mechanism knowledge.

Supervision next proceeds to the question of whether a youth is making clinical progress. The flow chart prioritizes the case history in the clinical reports to educate this decision. If a youth is making progress, continuation of the current treatment is recommended (regardless of whether it is a qualifying evidence-based service according to the general services research). If a youth is not improving, the appropriateness of the treatment selected is reconsidered. Case history (ie, clinical reports) and services research evidence (ie, evidence-based services reports) are prioritized for guiding this decision. If a treatment selection problem is identified, then the guidance recommends identifying relevant barriers using services research, local aggregate, and causal mechanism evidence and revising the treatment plan to select a more favorable intervention (Fig. 4).

If a youth is not improving despite the proper selection of an appropriate, evidence-based treatment, then the next decision concerns the quality or integrity of the treatment provided. This decision prioritizes the general services, local

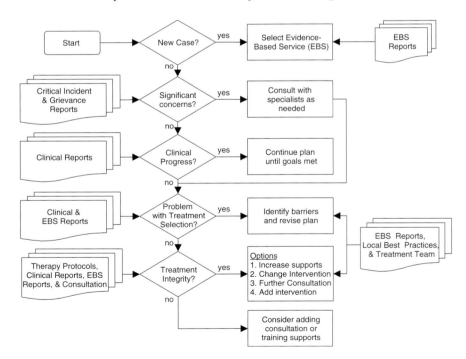

Fig. 4. Decision flow chart that models the Hawaii Child and Adolescent Mental Health Division's guidance for evidence-based clinical decision making.

aggregate, and case history evidence to review the specific practices that are part of the empirically based protocols, the practices that were part of other effective implementations in the local environment, and the practices that were used with the specific case in question. If problems with treatment quality or integrity are identified, then additional consultation or training is recommended to improve treatment quality and increase integrity. If no treatment integrity problems are identified, then a difficult situation is encountered: the best evidence-based treatments have been selected and implemented with high quality but have not helped the client sufficiently. At this point, evidence requirements may need to be relaxed and the "next best" evidence from all sources be applied to find interventions (eg, increase supports, change or add interventions, add additional experts) that hopefully will interact favorably with the client's circumstance to produce change.

Final illustration

One risk of such guided decision making is the potential for drift into micromanagement. A decision maker can turn quickly from feeling supported to feeling burdened by guidance. A related risk in the attempt to educate many decisions is that a system may become overburdened with data gathering. The cost of data gathering, analysis, and delivery must be weighed constantly against the realized benefit of improved decision making. CAMHD staff continually struggle with the temptation to gather relatively easy and inexpensive data without a clear and essential tie to decision making. This may paradoxically increase decision-making errors by creating "red herrings" and "cognitive noise."

The CAMHD system and its provider network have been working to strike a balance between providing sufficient guidance and oversight without micromanagement. Currently, providers maintain responsibility for the detailed, day-to-day service integrity and case monitoring (eg, daily phone surveys used with multidimensional treatment foster care [20], fear ratings used with cognitive-behavioral therapy for pediatric anxiety [21], and therapist adherence measures used with multisystemic therapy [3]), whereas the system maintains responsibility for providing less frequent, independent, standardized assessments of case progress, coordinating data, analyses, and decision guidance across providers, and managing intelligence related to general research and federal activities. The provider-to-system-level gap is spanned through the use of monthly treatment and progress summaries supplied by providers.

We conclude by providing an illustration of the synergy of this organization with respect to the treatment of depression using the CAMHD practice element codes [22]. Fig. 5 presents a comparison of the practice profiles obtained from (1) coding the general psychosocial services literature, (2) aggregated information from monthly provider summaries for youth with a

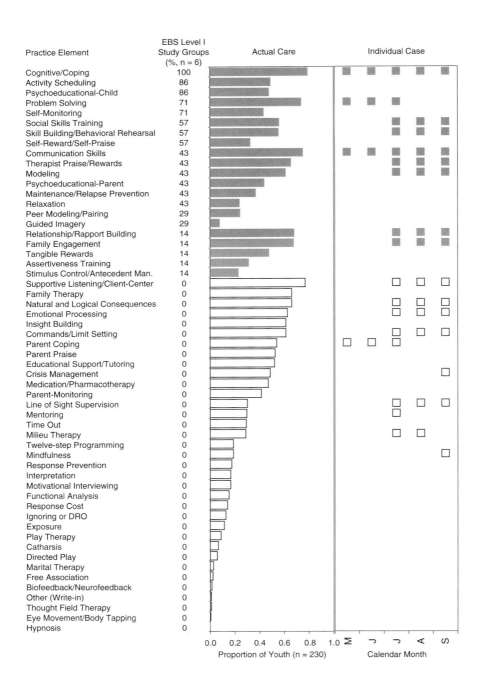

primary diagnosis of depression or dysthymia (actual care panel), and (3) historical information from the monthly provider summary for a specific case (case history). This type of analysis is insufficient to represent the moment-to-moment interactions between clinicians and clients, but from a quality review perspective, it may generate some interesting hypotheses about potential areas for performance improvement. For example, at first glance, the actual care panel indicates that not every youth in the system is currently treated with an evidence-based protocol. Many of the core practices incorporated in evidence-based protocols are implemented to some degree in the local care system, yet three of the five most commonly represented practices in the set of level I evidence-based protocols (ie, activity scheduling, child psychoeducation, and self-monitoring) were only used with roughly one half of cases in actual care. The open bars further indicate that many additional practices that were not included in the evidence-based protocols are used in the local care system. This may identify opportunities for improved efficiency through more focused interventions.

Examination of the individual case history follows a similar pattern. This youth's treatment began with several practices evident in the evidence-based protocols (ie, cognitive/coping, problem solving, communication skills) and included an additional practice element focusing on a parent's self-care (ie, parent coping). In the third month of treatment, intervention strategies became much more diffuse and included many additional practice elements that were and were not evidence based for depressed and withdrawn behavior. Other clinical reports required examination to understand the context associated with this proliferation, but this pattern and the inclusion of the milieu therapy and line of sight supervision elements is common in youth admitted to residential treatment (eg, related to suicidality). Taken together, it is clear that the observed treatment does not adhere closely to a single evidence-based protocol. Comparison of this individual case history to the aggregate actual care panel suggests that the treatment of the youth was fairly typical relative to similar youth in the local system. If the youth does not experience improvement with the current regimen and depressed or withdrawn behavior remains a target of treatment, the analysis identifies several evidence-based practices (ie, activity scheduling, child and parent psychoeducation, self-monitoring, self-reward, peer modeling, relaxation, guided imagery, assertiveness training, tangible rewards, stimulus control, and maintenance/relapse prevention) that might be considered as potential "next steps."

Fig. 5. Practice element profiles that illustrate the percent of study groups ($n = 6$) coded in the Hawaii evidence-based services literature review as qualifying in the category "Level 1 Best Support" for depressed or withdrawn behavior, the proportion of youth with a primary diagnosis of unipolar depression or dysthymia ($n = 230$) that actually received each practice element for one or more months during the fiscal year, and an individual case history that indicated whether each practice element was provided during each of five calendar months in the youth's treatment episode. Solid symbols identify practice elements that were included in at least one qualifying research study, and open symbols indicate practice elements that were not included in the qualifying studies.

Summary

This article described several of the strategies to promote and monitor the adoption of evidence-based decision making in Hawaii's system of care for youth. We identified several key clinical decisions that help focus our development efforts (ie, where and how a youth should be treated, whether the youth is receiving quality services, whether the youth is getting better, who should treat the youth, and how the youth's care should be supervised/managed). We specified the four evidence bases that may help educate these key decisions (ie, case history, local aggregate, general services research, and causal mechanism research). We introduced a few problems we encounter when we approach design from a treatment program versus treatment system perspective. We illustrated our efforts to deliver knowledge from the evidence bases to the key decision situations and described our struggle with the wisdom to guide prioritization among the evidence bases to keep from overwhelming decision makers.

This article discussed the Hawaii system of care's intensive engagement in the process of quality improvement but did not address whether these system reforms have yielded positive results for youth. The interested reader is referred to the performance reviews regularly published on the Child and Adolescent Mental Health Division Website [17,23]. In one notable analysis of the past 3 years, CAMHD [24] found evidence for a two- to threefold increase in the average monthly rate of improvement for youth as indexed by parent, teacher, and clinician reported measures of symptomatology and functioning. With many of the initial system reform goals achieved, new challenges have emerged. In the continual search for a better system, the CAMHD system may discard some of its current strategies, but one hopes that our future progress will continue to be guided by the best available evidence.

References

[1] Foster R, Groves I. Case-based review protocols. Tallahassee (FL): Human Systems and Outcomes; 1997.

[2] Chorpita BF, Yim LM, Donkervoet JC, et al. Toward large-scale implementation of empirically supported treatments for children: a review and observations by the Hawaii Empirical Basis to Services Task Force. Clinical Psychology: Science and Practice 2002;9:165–90.

[3] Henggeler SW, Schoenwald SK, Borduin CM, et al. Multisystemic treatment of antisocial behavior in children and adolescents. New York: Guilford; 1998.

[4] Mufson L, Moreau D, Weissman MM, et al. Interpersonal psychotherapy for depressed adolescents. New York: Guilford; 1993.

[5] Clarke G, Lewinsohn P, Hops H. Adolescent coping with depression course. Portland (OR): Kaiser Permanente Center for Health Research; 1990.

[6] Turk DC, Salovey P, Prentice DA. Psychotherapy: an information-processing perspective. In: Turk D, Salovey P, editors. Reasoning, inference, and judgment in clinical psychology. New York: Macmillan; 1988. p. 1–14.

[7] Chorpita BC, Daleiden E, Weisz JR. Identifying and selecting the common elements of evidence based interventions: a distillation and matching model. Ment Health Serv Res, in press.

[8] Whitley BE. Principles of research in behavioral science. 2nd edition. New York: McGraw Hill; 2002.

[9] Spiegler I. Knowledge management: a new idea or a recycled concept? Communications of the Association for Information Systems 2000;3:2–23.

[10] Child and Adolescent Mental Health Division. Evidence Based Services Committee: Biennial report. Hawaii Department of Health; 2004. Available at: http://www.hawaii.gov/health/mental-health/camhd/library/pdf/ebs/ebs-011.pdf. Accessed December 29, 2004.

[11] American Psychiatric Association. Diagnostic and statistical manual of mental disorders. 4th edition. Washington, DC: American Psychiatric Association; 1994.

[12] Achenbach TM, Rescorla LA. Manual for the ASEBA school-age forms and profiles. Burlington (VT): University of Vermont: Research Center for Children, Youth, and Families; 2001.

[13] Hodges K. Child and adolescent functional assessment scale (CAFAS). Ann Arbor (MI): Functional Assessment Systems; 1998.

[14] American Academy of Child and Adolescent PsychiatryAmerican Association of Community Psychiatrists. Child and adolescent level of care utilization system: user's manual. Washington, DC: American Academy of Child and Adolescent Psychiatry; 1999.

[15] Powsner SM, Tufte ER. Summarizing clinical psychiatric data. Psychiatr Serv 1997;48:1458–61.

[16] Kazdin A. Methodological issues and strategies in clinical research. Washington, DC: American Psychological Association; 1992.

[17] Hawaii Departments of Education and Health. Integrated performance monitoring reports. Hawaii Department of Health, 2004. Available at: http://www.hawaii.gov/health/mental-health/camhd/library/pdf/ipmr/index.html. Accessed December 29, 2004.

[18] Rogers EM. Diffusion of innovations. 4th edition. New York: Free Press; 1995.

[19] President's New Freedom Commission on Mental Health. Achieving the promise: transforming mental health care in America. Available at: http://www.mentalhealthcommission.gov/reports/reports.htm. Accessed December 29, 2004.

[20] Chamberlain P. Family connections: treatment foster care for adolescents with delinquency. Eugene (OR): Castalia Publishing; 1994.

[21] Kendall PC. Cognitive-behavioral therapy for anxious children: therapist manual. Ardmore (PA): Workbook Publishing; 1990.

[22] Child and Adolescent Mental Health Division. Instructions and codebook for provider monthly summaries. Hawaii Department of Health Child and Adolescent Mental Health Division. Available at: http://www.hawaii.gov/health/mental-health/camhd/pdf/paf/paf-001.pdf. Accessed December 29, 2004.

[23] Daleiden E. Annual evaluation report: fiscal year 2003. Hawaii Department of Health Child and Adolescent Mental Health Division. Available at: http://www.hawaii.gov/health/mental-health/camhd/library/pdf/rpteval/ge/ge002.pdf. Accessed December 29, 2004.

[24] Daleiden E. Child status measurement: system performance improvements during fiscal years 2002–2004. Hawaii Department of Health Child and Adolescent Mental Health Division. Available at: http://www.hawaii.gov/health/mental-health/camhd/library/pdf/rpteval/ge/ge010.pdf. Accessed December 29, 2004.

ELSEVIER
SAUNDERS

Child Adolesc Psychiatric Clin N Am
14 (2005) 351–366

CHILD AND
ADOLESCENT
PSYCHIATRIC CLINICS
OF NORTH AMERICA

Introducing and Evaluating Parent-Child Interaction Therapy in a System of Care

Eileen Franco, MPH[a,*], Robin E. Soler, PhD[a],
Mary McBride, PhD[b]

[a]*National Evaluation of the Comprehensive Community Mental Health Services for Children and Their Families Program, ORC Macro, 3 Corporate Square, Suite 370, Atlanta, GA 30329, USA*
[b]*Clackamas County Mental Health, Public Services Building, 2051 Kaen Road, Oregon City, OR 97045, USA*

Approximately 20% of all children and adolescents qualify for a "Diagnostic and Statistical Manual, edition 4" (DSM-IV) mental health diagnosis during the course of a year [1]. Approximately one half of these children display significant impairment that affects their ability to function in home, school, and the community. An even greater percentage of children and adolescents experiences subclinical behavioral and emotional problems. The Surgeon General's report on mental health [1] and the President's New Freedom Commission report on mental health [2] acknowledge that our nation's mental health service systems are not adequately addressing the mental health needs of children and adolescents. The New Freedom Commission directly addresses this problem by setting goals and providing recommendations for the transformation of the nation's mental health system. One goal specifically states that "excellent mental health care is delivered and research is accelerated" [2]. One of the recommendations made to the field encourages the dissemi-

---

Work on this article was supported by contract number 280-00-8040 with the Child and Family Branch of the Center for Mental Health Services (CMHS) in the Federal Substance Abuse and Mental Health Services Administration (SAMHSA).

* Corresponding author.
E-mail address: Eileen.Franco@orcmacro.com (E. Franco).

nation of evidence-based practices (EBPs), the evaluation of EBPs, and collaboration between private and public partners when implementing the "science
to practice" transfer of knowledge about EBPs and their implementation and
evaluation [2].

A growing body of knowledge exists about what works for children with
mental health needs [3]. Much of the research, however, has been conducted in
tightly controlled laboratory-based settings. There is a paucity of literature to
describe the experiences of service providers or service-providing agencies
as they work toward implementing EBPs or provide an understanding of
the effectiveness of EBPs in "real-world" settings. No research exists that ex-
amines the effectiveness of specific treatment modalities, such as EBPs, with
children with severe emotional disturbance who participate in comprehensive
mental health service systems (systems of care) such as those supported through
the federally funded Comprehensive Community Mental Health Services for
Children and Their Families Program [4–6]. The purpose of this article is to
describe the experiences of a service providing agency and an evaluation team
that is examining the effectiveness of an evidence-based treatment designed to
improve behavioral outcomes of children with a disruptive behavior disorder
who receive services in a system-of-care context.

In 1998, the Institute of Medicine (IOM) published a report on the state of
community-based drug and alcohol treatment programs [7]. The authors of the
report made a series of recommendations to promote the merging of practice
with research that directly applies to children's mental service research and
provision. These recommendations included supporting the development of
an infrastructure to facilitate research within a network of community-based
treatment programs, developing research initiatives to foster studies that include
community-based treatment programs as full partners, orienting research centers
and supporting structures to foster broad participation among researchers,
practitioners, consumers, and payers in the development of a treatment research
agenda, including studies to measure outcomes and program operations, and
cooperating in the development of financial incentives that encourage the
inclusion of proven treatment approaches into community-based treatment
programs [7]. The report also made recommendations regarding knowledge
development, dissemination and transfer, consumer participation, and training
to promote collaboration between researchers and communities.

In 2002, the Comprehensive Community Mental Health Services for Children and Their Families Program and the national evaluation contractors for
this program (referred to as the "national evaluation team") embarked on an
endeavor that directly responds to the recommendations of the President's New
Freedom Commission and the IOM report. Comprehensive Community Mental
Health Services for Children and Their Families Program and the national
evaluation team, with the support of the program's service evaluation work
group, provided the infrastructure and developed a process to transfer knowledge from the area of children's mental health research to the field of children's
mental health services. This collaboration resulted in the creation of the treat-

ment effectiveness study (TES). The TES included community-based mental health services systems as full partners in the selection, implementation, and evaluation of an EBP. A full-scale evaluation and treatment fidelity plan was developed, and funding was provided to ensure full and adequate training in the EBT and to support and maintain fidelity of the EBP.

The goal of the TES is to examine whether children who receive an evidence-based treatment delivered in a system-of-care experience have better outcomes and maintain those outcomes longer than children in the same system who do not receive the evidence-based treatment. The TES was designed to address the following research questions: (1) What additional effects on child and family outcomes does an EBT delivered in a system-of-care experience compared with system-of-care services as usually delivered? (2) Was the EBT implemented faithfully in accordance with treatment guidelines? (3) How well is the EBT integrated with other system-of-care services and features?

Although these core questions provided the structural framework for the evaluation and fidelity assessment of the EBT, the TES also provided an opportunity to obtain important information on "real world" implementation issues: (1) How community-based agencies and providers respond to EBTs. (2) How well community-based clinicians are able to adhere to a manualized treatment approach. (3) How well children and their caregivers adhere to treatment expectations. (4) How community-based factors impact implementation of EBTs.

What is a system of care?

Before embarking on a description of EBTs and the TES, it is important to understand the service context in which the TES was developed and implemented. In 1993, the Child and Family Branch of the Center for Mental Health Services in the Federal Substance Abuse and Mental Health Services Administration launched the Comprehensive Community Mental Health Service for Children and Their Families Program. The goal of this program was to establish or develop service systems for children with severe emotional disturbance that used a system-of-care philosophy as their base [8,9]. The system-of-care philosophy asserts that to serve children with serious emotional disturbance, service delivery systems must offer a wide array of accessible, community-based service options that center on children's individual needs, include the family in treatment planning and delivery, and are provided in a culturally competent manner. An emphasis is placed on serving children in the least restrictive setting that is clinically appropriate. Because many children with serious emotional disturbances use various services and have contact with several child-serving agencies, service coordination and interagency collaboration are critical. The philosophy holds that if services are provided in this manner, outcomes for children and families will be better than can be achieved in more traditional

service delivery systems. The TES study was conducted in two communities
that were funded through this federal effort.

Why evidence-based treatments?

The Comprehensive Community Mental Health Services for Children
and Their Families Program includes a congressionally mandated national
evaluation that has been conducted in grant communities since 1994. When
this evaluation was initiated there was significant interest in understanding
how services provided in communities funded to implement systems of care
compared with mental health services provided "as usual" or without the aid of
federal funding. Child and family-level change was of particular interest. Initial
quasi-experimental comparison studies that captured outcomes for children and
families in funded programs compared with children and families in non-funded
match communities resulted in a multitude of findings regarding the effectiveness of the system-of-care philosophy [10–13]. The results generated more
questions than they answered, which further emphasized the need to better
understand what works, for whom, and under what conditions within systems of
care. This finding coincided with an increasing trend in mental health services to
transport clinical practices developed and found effective in university-based
settings to the community. A paucity of research in this area helped support the
development of the study of evidenced-based treatments in federally funded
system-of-care grant communities.

Implementation of the treatment effectiveness study

Implementation of the TES involved a multistage process. The process was
initiated with a treatment nominations process [14]. Experts in the field of
children's mental health and mental health services were asked to nominate
clinical treatment modalities that proved effective in the reduction of emotional
or behavioral problems among children and met standard criteria for EBP [15].
Submitted nominations were reviewed and scored according to EBT criteria.
This process resulted in a list of 11 evidence-based treatments. Of these,
1 already was well studied in community-based settings, and the development
team was not available for consultation for another.

After completion of the nominations process, community selection and
recruitment were initiated. Two communities were selected from among
all system-of-care communities that received federal funding in 1998. Communities had to show relative success in their implementation of the system-
of-care philosophy as evidenced through the national evaluation system of
care assessment study, have the capacity to serve more than 100 children in
a 12-month period, and have an interest in including an EBT among their service

array. Communities also had to have somewhat different program goals and target populations and be based in different types of geographic settings.

The evidence-based treatment

Once communities were selected, a local treatment selection process ensued. Agency directors reviewed the list of EBTs selected through the nomination process and considered their local needs and child and family characteristics. Both communities selected parent-child interaction therapy (PCIT) [16]. PCIT is a therapeutic technique for children aged 3 to 9 who have a disruptive behavior disorder. PCIT combines the teachings of play therapy and cognitive behavior therapy and uses data-driven decision making to guide progress through the treatment program [16]. The goal of the therapy is to provide caregivers with an advanced set of skills and techniques to promote incidents of positive behaviors and reduce incidents of challenging behaviors. There are two components of PCIT (child-directed interaction and parent-directed interaction) that each include six modules. Most of these modules require the presence and participation of the caregiver and child, although two caregivers and occasionally siblings may participate. A module is typically completed in one session, but caregivers must show evidence that they are using specific PCIT techniques before advancing to the next module. Child-directed interaction, the component of PCIT that is first introduced to children and their caregivers, is similar to play therapy in that parents engage their child in a play situation with the goal of strengthening the parent-child relationship, whereas parent-directed interaction, the second component, resembles clinical behavior therapy in that parents learn to use specific behavior management techniques as they play with their child. PCIT has been examined extensively [16–20], and results have indicated less oppositional-defiant, conduct, and severe behavior problems among children who received PCIT compared with children in a wait-list comparison group and significant changes on parents' self-report of psychopathology, personal distress, and parenting locus of control [20,21]. Measures of consumer satisfaction in all studies have shown that parents are highly satisfied with the process and outcome of treatment at its completion [22,23].

Implementation of parent-child interaction therapy

Simpson [24] proposed a model of program change for introducing research in the drug treatment area to practice in community settings. This model incorporates an understanding of institutional and personal readiness, organizational dynamics, staff needs related to exposure to the practice and ultimate buy-in for practice, institutional support needs, and resulting organizational change and program improvement. There are four action steps included with in this framework: (1) exposure to the treatment (through various modes of training), (2) adoption or intent to try the treatment, (3) implementation, and (4) full practice or routine use of the practice. Within this model, factors that influence change include motivation, institutional resources, convenience, reception and use of the practice, organizational climate, availability of institutional supports, and staff attributes. A review of the literature on dissemination of EBTs for children [25] shows that a key factor in successful dissemination relates to provision of detailed manuals and thorough training models (stages 1 and 2 of the Simpson model).

Introduction of PCIT to the Clackamas County mental health system provided an example of the successes and challenges associated with introduction of a research-based practice to the field. When PCIT was selected by participating communities as the EBT to introduce and evaluate, a lead trainer and researcher in PCIT was contacted and a contractual relationship was developed to ensure full and adequate support and training. The trainer worked closely with the TES team on the implementation of the intervention and worked with the community-based providers assigned to the treatment condition.

The PCIT trainer provided three levels of training to each service provider. The national evaluation team, community-based agency, and lead trainer conducted an initial 4-day intensive training session. This training included a general overview of PCIT (which was open to agency representatives, caregivers, and other community members), detailed description of the goals of PCIT and therapeutic techniques used to meet these goals, overviews and practice with each module of PCIT, training in the language used to direct caregivers and assess progress in PCIT, and description of and practice with coding of parent-child interaction (the results of which are used to assist a clinician in determining when to move forward with the caregiver to the next treatment module).

Before the training, all service providers were provided a copy of "Parent-Child Interaction Therapy: A Step-by-step Guide for Clinicians" [16]. During the training, each service provider received manuals to support implementation with fidelity. One manual included a series of module guides with each step of the session described in detail. The second manual included (1) an overview of the study, (2) description of study procedures, (3) detailed session checklists (including abbreviated versions of each module guide) that served as a research fidelity tool, (4) session review forms for recording non-PCIT techniques used in PCIT sessions and techniques used in sessions in which PCIT was not the focus, and (5) supporting materials associated with PCIT goals and procedures that are given to caregivers. Service providers also were given a set of toys to use during the session (eg, construction toys, magic markers, a small doll house) and homework kits that included a few small items for children and their caregivers to use at home when practicing PCIT skills.

Each month during the course of the study (approximately 20 months), the PCIT trainer conducted PCIT fidelity consulting sessions. For these sessions, participants called a central conference line and discussed successes and challenges in the implementation process. Questions were addressed and responses to the questions were compiled into a PCIT "Frequently Asked Questions Guide" that was later distributed to all PCIT service providers.

The treatment effectiveness study evaluation design

The TES is part of a larger evaluation effort designed to assess the development and success of EBPs introduced to systems of care funded by the Center of Mental Health Services. This evaluation is comprehensive in scope and involves a study that serves to describe basic demographic characteristics of children served and their families and assesses a broad range of emotional, behavioral, educational, and child and family functioning outcomes and service use experiences. Data are obtained upon entry to the service system (or within 30 days of intake) and every 6 months thereafter (for up to 18 months in the case of the TES). These study components serve as the basis for the overall quantitative data collection component of this TES. Details of the national evaluation protocol are described elsewhere [4–6,14,26–28]. In addition to the national evaluation data collected, children were screened for attention deficit hyperactivity disorder, conduct disorder, and oppositional-defiant disorder through caregiver interviews using a computerized version of the Diagnostic Interview Schedule for Children (unpublished data). Outcomes related to PCIT are also assessed at 3-month intervals for a 1-year period (with a final data collection interview occurring at the 18-month data collection point). The Eyberg Child Behavior Inventory [29] and DSM–IV structured interview are administered to caregivers to assess disruptive behavior. Children and caregivers are also observed at intake and at the 6-month follow-up interview. These observations are coded using the didactic parent-child interaction coding system [30]. Fidelity of PCIT implementation is assessed using checklists administered to caregivers and clinicians, who evaluate the degree to which the clinicians adhere to the PCIT model. Exposure to other therapeutic techniques also is assessed with session review forms. Overall involvement in a broader array of services is assessed as part of the larger national evaluation protocol. Adherence to the system-of-care philosophy was assessed with a randomly selected subsample of the overall study population using the system-of-care practice review [31]. The protocol uses information drawn from a review of a child's mental health service agency records and a series of interviews with the caregiver, primary service provider, and informal provider to develop scores on domains that address different aspects of the system-of-care philosophy.

The TES used a randomized controlled trial design, which allows for the testing of the effects of the EBT integrated into the system-of-care approach versus system-of-care services as usual. There was an intervention group and a control group. Service providers in the treatment group received the training and materials described previously. In Clackamas County Mental Health (CCMH), random assignment occurred initially at the service provider level to receive PCIT training; subsequently children were randomized to a PCIT-trained therapist or a control therapist. Both groups that participated in the study in each community continued to be eligible for other system-of-care services. Service providers in the control group were given a general overview of the study and its goals, a set of session checklists, and the same types of toys provided for therapy sessions and homework kits, but no direction was given as to how to use the toys. The service providing agencies, the national evaluation team, and the PCIT trainer coordinate a PCIT training for all control group service providers after all children and their caregivers served have reached the 18-month data collection point.

Lessons learned in the real world

The evaluation team and CCMH staff learned many practical lessons about what it takes to implement an EBT. The lessons learned by evaluation team members and agency staff are similar in many ways but also are related directly to their needs and expectations. These similarities and differences emphasize the importance of the need for collaboration when implementing a successful evaluation for the EBT.

Lessons learned by the Clackamas County mental health system

Service providers and agencies often are put in the position of valuing and wanting to implement EBPs but find that there are few that fit the population being served. For example, many practices may be "promising" and attractive to a community, but the clinical trials that support the practice many have been conducted in a different setting than that in which the agency is based or with different age groups or with children and families who have a different diagnostic presentation than the agency's target population. Community-based mental health providers need EBPs that have shown clinical effectiveness in community-based settings. The Clackamas County mental health system embarked on this endeavor with the understanding that few, if any, EBPs existed that would be the needs of different sectors of its service population. They also had the shared goals of beginning to develop knowledge about what might work in their community for young children with disruptive behavior disorders.

The first lesson learned by agency staff was that participation in this complex study "is worth it." They quickly recognized that it takes (1) commitment at all levels of the agency from clinicians to managers, (2) repeated communication about the commitment made, and (3) willingness to change. Two major changes made by agency staff include the move to data-driven treatment decisions and development of performance expectations that support the use of EBPs.

Once CCMH fully bought into the study, many other challenges and opportunities for learning occurred. Agency staff learned the following lessons:

- There is an added time commitment at every level of implementation of PCIT and the evaluation of PCIT. Although "additional" time was allotted for each step of the process, it still took twice as long as planned.
- Management had to develop ways to facilitate clinician and family participation in the clinical trial. Every time a clinician or family faced a problem or what is perceived as a "barrier," it became the manager's responsibility to use the systems in place to become a true "barrier buster." Time and management skills are just two components of the infrastructure required to implement EBPs.
- To ensure fidelity, training is necessary for implementation of EBP. This training is essential, expensive, and never ending. At minimum, (1) the service-providing agency must plan for monthly updating and review of the clinical intervention being studied, (2) clinical supervisors must review cases over time to ensure that fidelity to the intervention model being studied is maintained, (3) use of fidelity checklists alone are not adequate to sustain the EBP, and (4) frequent supportive consultation among the clinical peers and managers must occur.
- Some families and staff had to experience a paradigm shift for successful implementation. Family involvement and family-driven service planning are core values and principles associated with the system-of-care philosophy. These values are also consistent with PCIT. PCIT is parent/child focused, however; it is not a child-centered treatment. PCIT is also a shorter term and intensive treatment. As a result, clinicians had to work toward developing long-term relationships with children and their families that were intermittent in intensity. This approach differs from the more traditional long-term child-focused treatment strategies that the staff were accustomed to using. Families had to shift their expectations and become more actively involved in their child's treatment. The option of leaving children at the door of the clinic and returning to pick them up after running errands was gone with PCIT. Not only did parents have to attend sessions in the clinic with their children but also they had homework assignments. Although these homework assignments were only 5 minutes long, for some families this was a major issue. Family engagement is crucial and challenging. PCIT requires an intensive time commitment, and often it was only after the families were partially into PCIT that they finally understood what they committed to and found it worth it.
- CCMH staff learned that they needed to maintain flexibility with service planning when implementation started. As with any group clinical intervention, some families needed to do some individual or focused work before starting PCIT. Sometimes PCIT had to be interrupted and suspended for a while because of crisis issues.

- Keeping interest and motivation of families to complete the intervention became a challenge for clinicians. CCMH staff found early on that reaching "mastery" with PCIT took longer than anticipated. Early clinical studies indicated that PCIT was a 12-session intervention model. In some cases, however, a session in a module actually took up to 3 weeks for a family to demonstrate "mastery."

- Clinicians traditionally have not been involved in research studies at CCMH. Many questions and concerns were raised initially about the methodology. Such struggles often were phrased in statements about "ethical" concerns that control clinicians were being asked to provide a "less adequate service" and treatment families who received PCIT were getting "favorite" status. In closely listening to the clinicians, the issues were basically grouped in two ways: (1) Clinicians were forgetting that PCIT was not yet an EBP for the Comprehensive Community Mental Health Services for Children and Their Families Program target population. (2) Clinicians were committed and struggling to "make it work." The issues of "favoritism" were related to their questions about their need to treat PCIT families differently to ensure their participation. Questions that arose included "Should I hold the more desirable appointment times for PCIT families?" "Should I be more lenient with PCIT families when they don't show, come late, or cancel a lot?" Discussing the issues and the rationale allowed clinicians to resolve their concerns.

- Being involved in a randomized, clinical trial study requires additional paperwork. Because the paperwork (mostly fidelity checklists) was in addition to existing agency paperwork, it felt huge. The development of a monitoring system and tracking for completion of clinicians' paperwork also is a major time commitment for managers.

- Maintaining fidelity to PCIT became an everyday issue. Staff were regularly reminded that maintaining fidelity was essential to having confidence in the findings generated. Part of the monitoring of fidelity included ensuring that there was not some "borrowing" of aspects of PCIT by control group clinicians. The more traditional way clinicians work is that they solicit input from each other and share resources of what they have found to work with families. Managers had to create a way to allow this exchange to continue for everything but PCIT.

- Motivation of the PCIT-trained clinicians happened through the successes and challenges they experienced with their families using PCIT. For the control therapists, however, the rewards had to be intrinsic, such as making the study successful or knowing that at the end of the study they would receive the same intensive training in PCIT that all treatment group clinicians received.

- Conducting this randomized clinical trial in the CCMH, a publicly funded community mental health center, brings many challenges to traditional researchers. CCMH experienced organizational changes caused by budget reductions that included office moves, staff turnover, administrative shuffles, and service delivery model changes, Despite these changes, CCMH continued their work with the study. These changes are part of the real world and are variables that must be identified and defined. They are not signs of failure or reasons to stop implementing EBPs or evaluating their effectiveness.

Lessons learned by the evaluation team

The national evaluation team, which is highly skilled and familiar with the clinical and behavioral characteristics of children with disruptive behavior disorders and the general functioning of systems of care, is, in the end, composed of evaluators with goals and expectations that coincide with the evaluation role. Working with CCMH and their staff under the direction of a local evaluation field coordinator provided many opportunities for understanding not only how effective PCIT might be but also how complex implementation of an EBT can be. Lessons learned by the national evaluation team include the following:

- Selecting an EBT that matches a community's needs and characteristics is a challenge in and of itself. Often, service providers look for the EBT that proves to be most effective in improving outcomes. The evaluation team learned that it is equally important to consider three main factors to ensure successful implementation, including (1) child and family characteristics, (2) service provider characteristics, and (3) resources available to facilitate implementation. Some child and family characteristics include family structure and stability, age of the child, cultural expectations that may run counter to the implementation plan, expectations about the therapeutic relationship, and availability of time. Service provider and agency characteristics include structure and stability of the agency, employment status and local laws and regulations around who can provide what types of service, general clinical skills, training background, therapeutic style, and openness to change. Resources include the obvious, such as funds for training and staff time, but also can be specific to the EBT itself. Laboratory-based implementation of PCIT requires the use of a two-way mirror, a designated play area, and a sound system that included a microphone and "bug" in the ear. These materials allow the child and caregiver to interact in a more naturalistic setting while the clinician "coaches" the caregiver to assist with the interaction. These resources were not available at CCMH agency offices. Adaptations were made, but it is unknown what impact these adaptations will have on the effectiveness of the intervention.
- Development of relationships between agency and evaluation staff is critical. The national evaluation team committed a full-time field coordinator, a deputy project manager, and a senior project manager to this study. The

team developed relationships with lead agency administrators, and the field coordinator worked closely with many different agency staff. The evaluation team addressed all questions and concerns of the care coordinator and clinicians related to the evaluation, and the PCIT trainer addressed details of PCIT implementation. The clinical supervision was centralized across the participating study clinicians and the lines of communication were clear. Participating care coordinators and clinicians were asked to modify their time and work. For example, clinicians must complete their session review form immediately after the session with the family, and care coordinators must complete the diagnostic (DISC) screening before assigning a clinician to the family.

- For a successful evaluation, it is necessary for the process of recruitment and enrollment to be seamless to service delivery. If multiple disruptions occurred in the day-to-day work of care coordinators and clinicians, they viewed the evaluation as a burden for themselves and the families and children they serve. Having the collaboration and support of program staff in leadership roles enabled local evaluators to have the needed support and leverage when challenges occurred. For example, if the local evaluation team was not getting compliance with completion of fidelity forms, the clinical supervisor reminded the clinician directly.

- Flexibility is key. CCMH faced several budget cuts and organizational restructuring. The clinical supervision structure of the study clinicians and the care coordinators changed. This change required development of new relationships. With restructuring, a few study clinicians and care coordinators were shifted to other roles, which reduced the number of people who were knowledgeable about the study. CCMH and the national evaluation team had to respond to these changes by shifting staff responsibilities, providing additional support to staff involved in the study, and ultimately, expanding the study completion date by a few months (to account for reduced enrollment that resulted for a decrease in staff availability).

- Random assignment created many challenges for CCMH. The national evaluation team had difficulty obtaining buy-in to the concept of random assignment from intake staff (ie, care coordinators) and families. As families received PCIT and the clinicians offered it, more people had interest in accessing that treatment option. It was viewed as cutting-edge treatment. Some care coordinators did not want to take the risk of enrolling a family into a study (and the family being selected for the control group) if they believed that the family would benefit from PCIT. Some families had the misperception that if they participated in the evaluation, they would only get PCIT and have no access to services offered within their system of care, although this was not true. The evaluation team had to educate staff and families when necessary. In addition to facing challenges of buy-in, random assignment had an impact on the cultural competency of the evaluation. A limited number of clinicians were bilingual. Monolingual Spanish-speaking youth and parents were not included in the evaluation. Because only one bilingual provider was available, random assignment into treatment or control conditions was not possible.

- Additional time is required for diagnostic screening. In accordance with the study design, the care coordinators administered the DISC to families during intake assessment. The screener ensured eligibility consistency across the communities in terms of the diagnostic information. Initially, administering the DISC required more time than expected. The care coordinators believed it was unfair to take the families' time without some type of compensation or incentive. Families were starting to perceive the DISC as the cause of delay in receiving services, which hindered enrollment into the evaluation. The evaluation team met these challenges in different ways. Further DISC training was provided to the intake staff to decrease the time for administration by increasing their familiarity with the instrument. Families were assured that services were not being delayed by participating in the study. A monetary incentive was offered to families who completed the DISC. Finally, an alternate screener was made available. Members of the evaluation team could administer the DISC if the intake staff had limited time. These solutions were helpful in increasing enrollment into the study.

- Assessment of fidelity must be easy. To assess the fidelity of the intervention, study clinicians were required to submit therapist session review forms. The treatment clinicians also submitted fidelity checklist and Eyberg Child Behavior Inventories. The evaluation team provided these forms to the PCIT clinicians in an easy-to-use manual that was divided by PCIT session. This manual also included handouts and instructions for the PCIT clinicians to use. The evaluation team noted that several clinicians were not completing or submitting their forms in a timely basis. The field coordinators sent e-mail reminders and made follow-up phone calls. If the problem persisted, the evaluation team would enlist the help of the program staff supervisors.

- Sometimes real-world implementation demands that changes be made to evaluation design. The evaluation needed to re-evaluate some of the data collection timelines. PCIT has 12 modules; however, the communities were reporting that families were taking longer to reach mastery at each session or were missing appointments. Initially, the study design included a second observational coding (Dyadic Parent-Child Interaction Coding System [DPICS]) 3 months after intake to services (to coincide with the anticipated end of PCIT, which was designed as a 12-week intervention). It became apparent early on, however, that few, if any, families would complete PCIT in 3 months. In some cases, fewer than half of the required sessions were completed in that time period. As a solution, the data collection timelines changed and DPICS observations were scheduled for 6 months after intake to allow for more time to complete PCIT or at least reach parent-directed interaction, the second part of PCIT.

- Proper training that is interactive and engaging helps improve fidelity of the EBT and increases the confidence of clinicians. Training must go beyond basic workshops. It requires having easy-to-use manuals that also can help data collection efforts and aid treatment fidelity. In addition to the initial training, clinicians received booster training and participated in monthly consultations with the trainer, which provided ample time for troubleshooting concerns that arose during implementation.

Summary

In an effort to increase the nation's understanding of how well EBTs work in community-based settings and, more specifically, in communities that apply a system-of-care philosophy, the national evaluation of the Comprehensive Community Mental Health Services Program collaborated with community-based mental health agencies. Evaluating and implementing an EBT greatly adds knowledge to the field and may help leverage future funding streams for communities. This article described a TES and outlined lessons learned by a participating community-based agency (CCMH) and the evaluation team. Many important lessons were learned, many of which were related to the impact of buy-in, training, and availability of resources on implementation of an EBT. Buy-in of program staff to implement the EBT and its evaluation helped achieve adherence to the treatment protocol, completion of fidelity forms, and commitment in motivating families to participate. Several resources are needed for implementation, including clinical supervision, office space, time, dedicated staff, and training. ORC Macro dedicated staff to conduct the evaluation (ie, a full-time field coordinator) and the PCIT training (ie, trainer) and provided manuals for clinicians. Clackamas County mental health staff tried to conserve resources for the EBT in the face of budget cuts and organizational changes. Overall, the complexity of real-world practice required significant commitment and flexibility.

Implementation of an EBT in a real-world setting is important and worth the effort. If a good plan is put in place for the EBT and its evaluation and the commitment of all program staff and families is present, the EBT will be implemented and evaluated successfully. Concerns that arise with implementation must be addressed and explored. Evaluators and program staff must be creative with their solutions while still maintaining the fidelity of the EBT. The lessons learned by the program staff and evaluation team highlight important considerations for others who attempt to implement an EBT in their community.

Acknowledgments

The authors wish to specially thank Wayne Holden for his input and review of this article and Stacy Johnson for all her efforts as the field coordinator of the study in Clackamas County, OR.

References

[1] US Department of Health and Human Services. Mental health: a report of the surgeon general. Rockville: US Department of Health and Human Services, Substance Abuse and Mental Health Services Administration, Center for Mental Health Services, National Institutes of Health, National Institute of Mental Health; 1999.

[2] New Freedom Commission on Mental Health. Achieving the promise: transforming mental health care in America. Final report. (DHHS Pub. No. SMA-03-3832.) Rockville: US Department of Health and Human Services; 2003.

[3] Burns BJ, Hoagwood K, editors. Community treatment for youth: evidence-based interventions for severe emotional and behavioral disorders. New York: Oxford University Press; 2002.

[4] Center for Mental Health Services. Annual report to Congress on the evaluation of the comprehensive community mental health services for children and their families program, 1999. Atlanta (GA): ORC Macro; 1999.

[5] Center for Mental Health Services. Annual report to Congress on the evaluation of the comprehensive community mental health services for children and their families program, 2000. Atlanta (GA): ORC Macro; 2000.

[6] Center for Mental Health Services. Annual report to Congress on the evaluation of the comprehensive community mental health services for children and their families program, 2001. Atlanta (GA): ORC Macro; 2001.

[7] Lamb S, Greenlick MR, McCarty D, editors. Bridging the gap between practice and research: forging partnerships with community-based drug and alcohol treatment. Washington, DC: National Academies Press; 1998.

[8] Stroul BA, Friedman RM. A system of care for children and youth with severe emotional disturbances. Revised edition. Washington, DC: Georgetown University Child Development Center, CASSP Technical Assistance Center; 1986.

[9] Pires S. Building systems of care: a primer. Washington, DC: Georgetown University Child Development Center; 2002.

[10] Brannan AM, Baughman L, Reed E, et al. System-of-care assessment: cross-site comparison of findings. Children's Services: Social Policy, Research, and Practice 2002;5:35–56.

[11] Stephens RL, Holden EW, Hernandez M. System-of-care practice review scores as predictors of behavioral symptomatology and functional impairment. Journal of Child and Family Studies, in press.

[12] Holden EW. Medication use for children in systems of care. Presented at the annual meeting of the American Psychiatric Association. Philadelphia, May 2002.

[13] Foster EM, Connor T, The public costs of better mental health services for children and adolescents. Psychiatr Serv, in press.

[14] Center for Mental Health Services. Annual report to Congress on the evaluation of the comprehensive community mental health services for children and their families program, 2002. Atlanta (GA): ORC Macro; 2002.

[15] Chambless DL, Hollon SD. Defining empirically supported therapies. J Consult Clin Psychol 1998;66(1):7–18.

[16] Hembree-Kigin TL, McNeil CB. Parent–child interaction therapy: a step-by-step guide for clinicians. New York: Plenum Press; 1995.

[17] Herschell AD, Calzada EJ, Eyberg SM, et al. Parent-child interaction therapy: new directions in research. Cognitive and Behavioral Practice 2002;9:9–16.

[18] Eyberg SM, Funderbunk BW, Hembree-Kigin TL, et al. Parent-child interaction therapy with behavior problem children: one and two year maintenance of treatment effects in the family. Child and Family Behavior Therapy 2001;23:1–20.

[19] Borrego Jr J, Urquiza AJ, Rasmussen RA, et al. Parent-child interaction therapy with a family at high risk for abuse. Child Maltreat 1999;4:27–54.

[20] Schuhmann EM, Foote R, Eyberg S, et al. Parent-child interaction therapy: interim report of a randomized trial with short-term maintenance. J Clin Child Psychol 1998;27:34–45.

[21] Nixon DV, Sweeney L, Erickson DB, et al. Parent-child interaction therapy: a comparison of standard and abbreviated treatments for oppositional defiant preschoolers. J Consult Clin Psychol 2003;71(2):251–60.

[22] Brestan EV, Eyberg SM, Boggs SR, et al. Parent-child interaction therapy: parents' perceptions of untreated siblings. Child and Family Behavior Therapy 1997;19(3):13–28.

[23] Eisenstadt TH, Eyberg S, McNeil CB, et al. Parent-child interaction therapy with behavior problem children: relative effectiveness of two stages and overall treatment outcomes. J Clin Child Psychol 1993;22(1):42–51.

[24] Simpson DD. A conceptual framework for transferring research to practice. J Subst Abuse Treat 2002;22:171–82.

[25] Herschell AD, McNeil CB, McNeil DW. Clinical child psychology's progress in disseminating empirically supported treatments. Clinical Psychology: Science and Practice 2004;11:267–88.

[26] Holden EW, Friedman RM, Santiago RL. Overview of the national evaluation of the comprehensive community mental health services for children and their families program. Journal of Emotional and Behavioral Disorders 2001;9:4–12.

[27] Manteuffel B, Stephens R, Santiago R. Overview of the national evaluation of the comprehensive community mental health services for children and their families program and summary of current findings. Children's Services: Social Policy, Research, and Practice 2002;5(1):3–20.

[28] Vinson N, Brannan AM, Baughman L, et al. The system-of-care model: implementation in twenty-seven communities. Journal of Emotional and Behavioral Disorders 2001;9:30–42.

[29] Eyberg S, Pincus D. Eyberg child behavior inventory and Sutter-Eyberg student behavior inventory, revised professional manual. Odessa (FL): Psychological Assessment Resources, Inc.; 1999.

[30] Eyberg SM, Bessmer J, Newcomb K, et al. Dyadic parent-child interaction coding system. II: A manual. Soc Behav Sci Documents (Ms. No. 2897). San Rafael (CA): Select Press; 1994.

[31] Hernandez M, Gomez A, Lipien L, et al. Use of the system-of-care practice review in the national evaluation: evaluating the fidelity of practice to system-of-care principles. Journal of Emotional and Behavioral Disorders 2001;9:43–52.

ELSEVIER
SAUNDERS

Child Adolesc Psychiatric Clin N Am
14 (2005) 367–370

CHILD AND
ADOLESCENT
PSYCHIATRIC CLINICS
OF NORTH AMERICA

Index

Note: Page numbers of article titles are in **boldface** type.